A STUDY OF DOCTORS

TAVISTOCK

The International Behavioural and Social Sciences Library

HEALTH & SOCIETY
In 12 Volumes

A STUDY OF DOCTORS

Mutual Selection and the Evaluation of Results in a Training Programme for Family Doctors

MICHAEL BALINT, ENID BALINT,
ROBERT GOSLING AND
PETER HILDERBRAND

First published in 1966 by
Tavistock Publications Limited

Reprinted in 2001 by
Routledge
2 Park Square, Milton Park, Abingdon, Oxon, OX14 4RN

Transferred to Digital Printing 2007

Routledge is an imprint of the Taylor & Francis Group

© 1966 Michael Balint, Enid Balint, Robert Gosling
and Peter Hildebrand

British Library Cataloguing in Publication Data
A CIP catalogue record for this book
is available from the British Library

A Study of Doctors
ISBN 0-415-26425-1
Health & Society: 12 Volumes
ISBN 0-415-26509-6
The International Behavioural and Social Sciences Library
112 Volumes
ISBN 0-415-25670-4

A Study of Doctors

MUTUAL SELECTION AND THE EVALUATION
OF RESULTS IN A TRAINING PROGRAMME
FOR FAMILY DOCTORS

MICHAEL BALINT, ENID BALINT,
ROBERT GOSLING & PETER HILDEBRAND

TAVISTOCK PUBLICATIONS

J. B. LIPPINCOTT COMPANY

First published in Great Britain in 1966
by Tavistock Publications Limited
2 Park Square, Milton Park, Abingdon, Oxon, OX14 4RN
in 11 point Times New Roman
by Butler & Tanner Ltd, Frome

Distributed in the United States of America
and Canada by J. B. Lippincott Company,
Philadelphia and Montreal

Contents

Contents

Introduction

EVERY year all over the Western world more and more post-graduate courses are organized for general practitioners offering them training in some sort of psychiatry or psychotherapy. This is true not only in the United Kingdom, but also in France, Holland, Germany, Switzerland, and the United States.

A superficial survey might suggest that there is nothing special in this development: psychiatry is a developing field in medicine and so it is only natural that more and more doctors should be interested in it. Closer scrutiny, however, reveals that there is a significant difference between these courses and all the others. Although in the field of undergraduate education many critical studies have been made of the effectiveness of the courses offered, in the postgraduate field the adequacy of the teaching for general practitioners is more or less taken for granted with one clear exception, namely, the teaching of psychiatry and psychotherapy. The authorities subsidizing or organizing these courses seem to have serious doubts about the value of this sort of training. This is especially true in the United States where there are in progress various research projects which aim at evaluating their efficiency.

This is surprising indeed. Apparently nobody has ever questioned the real efficiency of the refresher courses for general practitioners in cardiology, paediatrics, rheumatology, the treatment of cancer, etc. Why is it that these questions are asked exclusively with regard to courses in psychiatry? Of course, there are many reasons for this difference; some are well known, but by tacit agreement are treated with silence or referred to only in passing. The aim of our research has been to highlight some of the reasons for this difference, to bring out some of the underlying problems, and, as far as our material allows, to propose some answers.

It is true that there is as yet no agreement about the sort of psychiatry needed in general practice. As a rule, however, the fact that experience has shown that so-called 'academic' or 'non-dynamic' psychiatry is of very limited use in this setting is glossed over. In addition, as our figures show, the fact that a psychiatrist has obtained a specialist qualification and a consultant post in a hospital is no guarantee that he will prove to be a successful teacher of general practitioners. In other words, we rediscovered the simple truth – that one must learn how to be a teacher. Further, we have good evidence that not every general practitioner, no matter how successful he has been in his profession, is a suitable candidate for training in psychological understanding and psychotherapeutic skill.

Our book is a critical examination of this complex problem, and we hope that in it the reader will find some answers. The reader must, however, be prepared to find in addition a number of unexpected problems. This is the fate of every research. When we clarify one problem by making the questions more precise so that a partial answer may be found, we are forced to realize our limitations and this helps us to discover problems that were previously hidden.

To present our findings in this volume, our plan has been to start with a description of the history of the training scheme and its socio-psychological structure, and then, in Chapter

x

3, to show why a selection procedure had been introduced. In order to assess the efficiency of our training method in general and the results of our selection procedure in particular, we had then to devise and apply a rating scale; the principles and reliability of the scale are described in Chapters 4 and 5, and the statistical results obtained with it in Chapters 6 and 7. Finally, in Chapter 8, our findings are summarized.

Although each chapter was thoroughly discussed by the whole research team, and thus the views expressed in this book are those held by us jointly and severally, it was decided that each chapter should be signed by the one who was responsible for its drafting. We hope that in this way the individuality of each contributor will come through more clearly and will make the book more varied and perhaps more interesting.

This Introduction concludes with a brief description of the roles of the four contributors in the training scheme.

Michael Balint, after making some abortive attempts in Budapest before 1939, started his first general practitioner seminar in London in the autumn of 1950 and has been engaged in this project ever since. In 1961, on retirement from the Tavistock Clinic, he joined the staff of the Department of Psychological Medicine at University College Hospital, London, where, in addition to running seminars for general practitioners, he has been trying to adapt this method to the training of medical students.

Enid Balint was the founder and the moving spirit of the Family Discussion Bureau. It was for this group of social workers that she and Michael Balint jointly worked out the training method which later was adapted for the purposes of training general practitioners. From the start she took part in this new venture, first as an associate-leader and case-supervisor, and in the last few years as the leader of a research seminar of general practitioners.

Robert Gosling was one of the first staff members of the Tavistock Clinic to join the team and so has seen the development of the training scheme from the last years of the pre-selection period onwards. Soon after joining he began to lead seminars of his own. For the two years before Michael Balint's retirement from the Tavistock Clinic he was jointly responsible for the developing training scheme and since then has been the tutor-in-charge. Recently, with P. M. Turquet, he has been engaged in writing a book on the dynamics of small groups as they affect the training of professional workers in seminars.

Peter Hildebrand, a consultant psychologist and psychoanalyst, became interested in the socio-psychological aspects of our training method and was invited to join our research team. At present, with J. L. Wilson, he is engaged in investigating the training process within a seminar of general practitioners.

CHAPTER 1

History *by* Robert Gosling

1. THE TAVISTOCK CLINIC

For the first dozen years after its foundation in 1920, the Tavistock Clinic was chiefly engaged in introducing into civilian practice experience in the new dynamic psychology gained during the First World War. It attempted to provide systematic psychotherapy for patients suffering from psychoneurosis and allied disorders. This attempt has had at least three results. First, it has focused interest on how the individual's personal resources have come to be what they are; how the vicissitudes of experience have moulded the innate endowment; and hence how child rearing influences mental health. Second, it has drawn attention to the varied ways in which these personal resources are invested in the environment, particularly the human environment, and how in turn the environment develops some and restricts others; this had led to an emphasis on group psychology and social psychiatry. And third, it has made it painfully obvious that the number of psychiatrists trained to undertake psychotherapy is, and will be for a very long time, far too small to meet the demand for individual attention.

Since about 1932, therefore, over and above therapeutic endeavours directly with patients, the staff of the Clinic has

1

devoted more and more of its time to the dissemination of psychological knowledge and skills to other professional workers of many kinds. To begin with this was done chiefly by using such traditional teaching methods as lectures and seminars. After the Second World War, however, the staff of the Tavistock Clinic and its newly founded associate institution, the Tavistock Institute of Human Relations, became intensely interested in the structure and function of groups. Some of those joining the staff after the war had in the Armed Forces been actively engaged in the use of small groups in selection procedures and rehabilitation. They now extended this interest to the exploration of groups as they exist in the community, such as marriages, families, and factories, and of small groups specially assembled for particular purposes, such as those for psychotherapy and those for training (Bion, 1961). This interest has had two important results: it has emphasized the central position of the family in studying and influencing mental health, and it has led to a much more deliberate use of the group dynamics of a seminar for the purpose of increasing professional skills. Thus over the years there has developed a considerable programme for the advanced training of professional workers directly concerned with the family, be they general practitioners, maternity and child welfare officers, paediatricians, social workers, probation officers, or some other.

This book is devoted to a short survey and evaluation of one such training scheme. It describes how the resources of the Tavistock Clinic have been deployed in the field of general practice in such a way as to spotlight psychological issues in this kind of work and at the same time to enable general practitioners to become more skilled in dealing with them. The scheme has evolved slowly over the past fourteen years (August 1950–January 1964), and while the plethora of variables at work makes rigorous evaluation impossible, a careful scrutiny of its development may reveal useful information.

2. ORIGINS OF THE SEMINARS FOR GENERAL PRACTITIONERS

In 1947 Enid Balint, working under the auspices of the Family Welfare Association, sought the help of the Tavistock Institute of Human Relations and the Tavistock Clinic in developing techniques for assisting people in marital difficulties and developing methods for training social workers in the use of these techniques. A seminar of social workers was formed for this purpose in 1948 and was named the Family Discussion Bureau. Early in 1949 Michael Balint was asked to join them. Enid and Michael Balint's collaboration resulted in the development of the 'case discussion seminar', which is still today the pivot of the work of the Family Discussion Bureau and which has been taken over for basic training in psychological understanding for a number of other professions. The main idea behind this method came from the way case-supervision had been integrated into psycho-analytic training in Hungary.

The special feature of the Hungarian psycho-analytic training was that the first case treated by the trainee was supervised by the trainee's own analyst. In this kind of supervision, instead of attention being paid exclusively to the patient's psychopathology and to the psychodynamics of the case, a certain amount was also paid to the interplay between the patient's transference and the trainee's counter-transference. This arrangement naturally led to a spreading of interest from the patient's material and psychopathology to the trainee's own emotional responses to it, and hence it led to an emphasis on the analyst–patient relationship as a two-way process. When Michael Balint then came to lead a

3

seminar of social workers concerned with marital difficulties it became clear to him that ordinary didactic methods were of very limited value; it also became clear to him, however, that if in the case discussion attention was focused on the developing client–worker relationship, a very considerable increase in the worker's understanding and effectiveness often resulted. A description of the subsequent work of the Family Discussion Bureau is to be found in several of their publications (Family Discussion Bureau, 1955, 1960, 1962).

Michael Balint had already used a similar approach with general practitioners in some experimental seminars during the 1930s when he was still in Hungary. Now, encouraged by its success with social workers in their handling of marital problems, he proposed to the Tavistock Clinic that he should again try this method with general practitioners. The Tavistock Clinic supported this proposal and in the autumn of 1950 the first seminar began.

3. THE FIRST SEMINAR

For some years it had been a frequent complaint of general practitioners that the training they had received at medical school for the care of their organically ill patients, though essential, had left them ill prepared for much of the work they were constantly called upon to do. They found that emotional difficulties of one kind or another were present, and were relevant, in a large proportion of their cases, but that they had no professional training in how to approach them. Along with many other hospital psychiatric departments, the Tavistock Clinic had attempted to make good this deficiency by offering postgraduate lectures or refresher courses from time to time. They had had the familiar rather disappointing result for all concerned: the student discovered how clever, or stupid, the psychiatrist was on his own ground,

4

but he gained very little that really prepared him better as a family doctor for his next encounter with a distressed patient in the middle of a busy surgery, with a worried mother when about to leave after an 'unnecessary' home visit, or with a patient exhibiting repeated minor ailments and signs of an unsatisfactory marriage in the background.

So what Balint proposed was to bring together a few general practitioners and psychiatrists for an extended period for the purpose of looking more realistically into the nature of the emotional turmoils into which a general practitioner is drawn if he is willing to notice them, and into the personal and professional resources actually available for dealing with them. An advertisement was therefore placed in the medical press announcing a 'Discussion Group Seminar on Psychological Problems in General Practice', and invitations were issued to a few doctors who had already shown an interest in psychological matters by attending a recent refresher course at the Clinic. Michael Balint was joined at the beginning of the first seminar by another member of the staff of the Clinic as co-leader. During the subsequent fourteen years there have been many developments in the training scheme and by January 1964 223 family doctors had taken part.

At the start, the assembled doctors, both general practitioners and psychiatrists, had to find out how they could work together, and along what lines. Inevitably there were clashes of aims and personalties and several doctors, including the co-leader, left feeling for one reason or another that the way the seminar was going was not one they wished to follow for a prolonged period. In fact, of the thirty-six general practitioners who joined in these early days only twenty-nine attended regularly; of these nine left after the first term, five after the second, and only fifteen stayed for any length of time. Two other psychiatrists joined the scheme temporarily, but likewise did not find it congenial. By 1952, however, there had emerged a group of doctors who had established enough of a common aim and who found the atmosphere of the seminars sufficiently congenial to make working together profitable. A lively sense of companionship and of breaking new ground together developed. They were organized by Michael Balint into a research team and became known as the 'Old Guard'. It was their joint work that formed the basis of our training method and that provided the material for Balint's book *The Doctor, His Patient and The Illness* (Balint, 1957a). The seminar stimulated and absorbed a great deal of the participants' interest and it remained completely stable in its composition for two and a half years.

Other psycho-analysts joined as associates for varying periods and some later contributed to the enterprise by offering a concurrent course of lectures for the exposition of psychodynamic theory. In 1953 another seminar was started under the leadership of one of them, but by common consent it was ended after two terms and only one member of it came back later for further training. For a time, as an experiment, those who wanted individual supervision of cases in addition to the discussions in the seminar were offered it by members of the Clinic staff; this practice was later abandoned as unprofitable. Another and more successful experiment was that of emergency consultations: after a thorough discussion in the seminar, and only if there was general agreement, the case was seen by a Clinic psychologist and psychiatrist who had then to report their findings back to the seminar for final evaluation. These emergency consultations have been used to a varying extent by different seminar leaders over the course of time.

Through all this period many approaches were explored by Balint and his 'Old Guard' and there was much trial and error. Gradually, as some lessons were learned, there

6

emerged the outline of a picture of what could be expected and what could profitably be done given the existing resources of the doctors concerned. The emergence of this picture – our training scheme – was signalled by the publication of the first paper in a professional journal (Balint, 1954), and resulted in Balint beginning to organize material for his book. Soon afterwards two new seminars were started, in October 1954 and April 1955, with the aim of testing out the new training methods, and there resulted in 1955 and 1956 the publication of six papers by various participants on experiences gained in the seminars (1955: Balint (2), Hopkins; 1956: Hopkins (2), Horder and others). In the following year two papers appeared in addition to Balint's book (1957: Balint, Saville). Between 1958 and 1960 there were nineteen papers published, and a public correspondence began concerning issues raised by this novel approach (1958: Abrahams (2), Clyne, Hopkins (2), Pasmore; 1959: Balint, Hopkins (3), Horder, Pasmore; 1960: Balint (3), Clyne (3), Hopkins).

The decision to start a new seminar in 1954 began a period of expansion of the training scheme that can be seen in the growth curve (*Figure 1*, p. 8). After a life of three years, what remained of the 'Old Guard' was reconstituted. Part of it formed the nucleus of a new seminar which aimed at providing a permanent forum for the discussion of particularly difficult or interesting cases by doctors who had already had some years of training; as old members have retired from it new ones have joined after a preliminary training period in other seminars, and to this day (1965) it continues. The other part of the 'Old Guard', together with a few doctors from the newer seminars were organized by Balint to undertake research into particular aspects of general practice. Their work has resulted in various publications. (Clyne, 1961, 1964; Clyne, Hawes, Lask, and Saville, 1963; Lask, in press).

7

A Study of Doctors

4. THE TRAINING SCHEME

Gradually, as the picture of what could be done in seminars of this type became clearer, all concerned began to orient themselves towards it and so the character of the seminars themselves began to be affected. General practitioners in the field now began to have some information, sketchy as it might be, of what they could expect from joining such a seminar. They read or heard of the kind of thing that went on and accordingly they made up their minds whether to apply to join or

FIGURE 1. DOCTORS TAKING PART IN THE TRAINING SCHEME

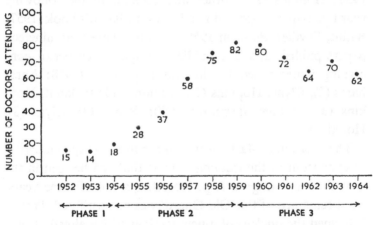

The construction of this graph is described on p. 19.

not. Formerly all that the prospective candidates had had to go on were the professed aims of the leader and the personalities of those involved. Now applicants had more detailed and explicit information available. This had an influence on the kinds of applicant coming forward: no longer was there such a premium on their being adventurers. The picture of what had been done in the past influenced the aims and expectations of new members. The Scheme became known less for its research component and more for its training; it

8

became more frequently referred to as 'A Course for General Practitioners' and sometimes even as 'Classes'.

During the period of expansion (see *Figure 1*) newcomers to the Scheme were not all general practitioners. As Balint's efforts began to show results, the Tavistock Clinic began to allow more and more of its staff to engage its time in this Training Scheme. During 1956 and 1957 three members of the staff began to attend the seminars regularly to learn something of the training technique that had been evolved so far, and later they started seminars of their own. The expansion, moreover, was not confined to the Tavistock Clinic. Four members of the staff of the Cassel Hospital, Richmond, attended for a period, and some of them later started seminars at their own hospital. A psychiatrist who had joined the 'Old Guard' and had provided theoretical lectures for it, and was later appointed to the staff of the University of Leeds, eventually established two seminars there for local general practitioners. Likewise a staff member from Canada took back something of his experience in the Scheme when he returned home, and a visitor from a mental hospital in London started his own seminar there after a period with us.

There also began at this time a considerable influx of visitors from other parts of the United Kingdom and from abroad, particularly from the United States, Holland, and Germany, and, more recently, from France and Switzerland. Though some were general practitioners, the majority were psychiatrists who were considering starting some similar activity in their home towns. A few have stayed to make an intensive study of the technique that has been evolved; the majority have had a more fleeting contact.

Thus information about the seminars has been distributed by way of articles and correspondence in the medical press, books deriving from the work of the seminars, visits on the part of interested outsiders, dispersal of trained personnel to

9

other parts, lectures given by participants to medical socie-
ties, and much informal discussion between colleagues. In
this way a public image that at first depended almost entirely
on fantasy has gradually been modified through the spread of
information.

By September 1958 there had accumulated a considerable
number of doctors who had had a preliminary period of
training and who now wanted to consolidate their gains or to
go further. How best to accommodate these doctors with
different ambitions and different abilities had then to be
considered. It was decided to try to provide two streams for
more advanced training, one for the fast and one for the
slow developers. The results of this step were inconclusive;
in addition, the staff were divided as to whether such a sorting
of the sheep from the goats provided a desirable model for
general practitioners who have themselves to give a service
to both 'good patients' and 'bad patients' alike. Latterly the
composition of seminars for advanced training has depended
more on trying to give doctors a variety of experience by
introducing them to colleagues who are new to them, than
in providing a seminar of a fairly uniform standard of work.
This question remains unsettled and still under consideration.

By this time also the number of staff members engaged in
this Scheme had become sufficiently large to warrant regular
meetings for technical discussions. These meetings have
grown in size as more psychiatrists have either started seminars of their own, or have attended regularly as participant
observers in preparation for undertaking leadership. Since
1961 they have taken the form of the detailed scrutiny of a
verbatim transcript of a seminar and a lively discussion of
the technical problems presented in it and the particular
leader's way of meeting them. In the course of time a fairly
wide variety of technical issues has been reviewed together
with several different ways of tackling them and the

results that ensue. These discussions on the technique of leadership were pursued on a wider front at two small international conferences devoted to this topic, the first at Brighton in 1962 and the second at Versailles in 1964, when psychiatrists attended from France, Germany, Holland, North and South America, and the United Kingdom.

In November 1959 a Conference was called for the purpose of evaluating the Training Scheme by the hundred or so doctors who by then had had direct experience of it. This was also attended by Dutch colleagues who had been engaged in a somewhat similar training scheme. The discussion and argument that resulted threw into relief some of the practical issues attendant upon such a training scheme and so helped to sharpen the self-image still further.

Just as the emergence of a picture of the work done in the seminar has changed the types of doctor coming forward to join them, so also has it affected the psychiatrist's behaviour. One particular way in which experience in the Training Scheme has been fed back into it by way of the psychiatrist's behaviour is in the introduction of a Mutual Selection Interview. Although the practice of advertising a proposed new seminar in the medicial press has been followed throughout, as more and more information became available, either by the written word or by hearsay, about what the seminars did, so the element of self-selection was affected. In addition, however, it had been found that using the particular technique developed by the original seminar under the leadership of Balint some doctors throve more than others, and some could make no use of it at all. This information was then used in a selection interview to modify still further the results of self-selection.

Surveying the personalities of the various doctors who had left the seminars prematurely by 1955 Balint had isolated three groups with fairly recognizable characteristics. He then

11

devised an initial interview intended both to enable the psychiatrist to recognize the doctor who was a poor risk and at the same time to enable such a doctor to realize that he would not find it easy to accept the aims and methods of the seminar (see Chapter 3). In this interview an attempt is made to see how good the fit is between the doctor's personality, expectations, and predilections on the one hand, and the sort of experiences that seminars of this kind seem to offer on the other. If the fit seems to be good, both parties to the interview feel fairly contented and the applicant is accepted. If the fit seems to be bad, either one or both together may decide to carry the matter no further.

For the first two years after the Mutual Selection Interviews were introduced, they were conducted by the psychiatrist into whose seminar the applicant would eventually go if he in fact joined the Scheme. Beside their personal experience and bias the psychiatrists were guided to some extent by the formulations that had been made by Balint. Since 1959 most of the interviews have been conducted by one psychiatrist, Gosling, as by that time the Scheme had grown to such a size that an officer, a tutor-in-charge, was needed to keep up with the routine administration.[1] It was at that time that the growth curve reached its plateau (*Figure 1*, p. 8).

From then until the end of our review period (1964) the growth curve has shown little change. The number of seminars and the total number of participants have remained more or less constant. The number of new applicants who have been accepted has remained at about twenty a year, and this has about matched the number leaving either prematurely or after three or four years of training. While the

[1] From 1959 to Balint's retirement in 1961 responsibility for administering the Scheme was divided between Balint and Gosling. Since then it has devolved upon the latter, while the former has been appointed to the staff of University College Hospital, London, where he has started some similar seminars.

12

growth curve indicates that a stable period has been reached, there has in fact been an increase in the number of psychiatrists undertaking prolonged study of this training technique. In addition to this increase in numbers of staff, however, there has also been an important qualitative change in that they were joined in 1961 by a consultant psychologist, Hildebrand, whose job it has been to take part in seminars and in technical discussions and to participate in research projects. Thus, while total numbers have latterly not changed greatly, there have been some important shifts of emphasis within the Scheme. One result of this period is the publication of this book; other results have yet to declare themselves.

CHAPTER 2

Structural Aspects of the Tavistock Training Scheme *by* Peter Hildebrand

1. FACTORS AFFECTING THE INITIAL STRUCTURE OF THE SCHEME: COMPARISON OF STRUCTURES

In this chapter I describe the development of the General Practitioner Training Scheme in socio-psychological terms. By adding this approach to the historical account given in Chapter 1 we highlight developments and conflicts in the Scheme and in our thinking which might otherwise have remained hidden.

I have attempted to develop a model of the Scheme as a social institution with a structure and a culture which are unique. The development of these features is difficult to define historically since the aims of the participants in the Training Scheme were kept ill defined, and clear-cut criteria for success or failure of the Scheme were not stated. In particular since there was no planned feed-back mechanism it was difficult for the results of the Training Scheme to influence training methods. My colleagues considered that this state of affairs was due in part to the importation into a training programme of the therapist's attitude, namely one of expectancy and open-mindedness with regard to what the final outcome may be.

14

It is noteworthy that in the treatment situation the result is generally arrived at only after a number of preferred alternatives have been explored and have been found to be inadequate by the patient. While effective ways of behaviour are being discovered, at the same time a certain amount of painful disillusionment is inevitable. In the treatment situation, the substitution of one set of aims for another, the giving up of beliefs in magical solutions, the idealization of the therapist, and the ending of treatment are all topics of concern and discussion.

On the other hand in a training scheme, secret aims and hopes may remain secret for the participants. The development of psychological skills may be deferred when an ending to the training period is postponed into the indefinite future. Where the seminar itself seems able to ignore both time and achievement, it is hard for its members to develop the sense of reality that would allow a proper assessment of skills in the light of experience. With no agreed period for the ending of training, doctors are given little impetus to assess themselves realistically and to change accordingly. Likewise, the staff can avoid any real validation of their techniques on the basis of results.

At the very least these attitudes and the structure which they engender make it very difficult to assess our scheme. In this it differs greatly from classical training schemes such as secondary and technical education, or University and professional training, in which all parties agree that the granting of a degree or diploma is the criterion of success. Here it is easy enough to work out the proportion of those who fail against those who succeed in gaining the qualification. Similarly, it is not difficult to lay down minimal requirements for entry and to exclude those applicants who, for one reason or another, do not meet them.

A second type of training – the postgraduate refresher

15

course for medical practitioners – generally has the aim of extending the doctor's factual knowledge and acquainting him with the developments or discoveries in a particular medical or surgical speciality. Any qualified practitioner may apply, and when he leaves after a short period, he will take with him such information as he can acquire according to his receptivity, acumen, and abilities. Generally, there is no formal attempt to evaluate the success of the refresher course in imparting the desired knowledge, and as long as the practitioner attends and pays his fee, all parties are presumed to be satisfied. The work is based on the teaching model and the distinction between teacher (consultant) and pupil (practitioner) is maintained. In these two types of training the work is either evaluated by the number of successes in gaining the desired diploma or no attempt is made to evaluate the work at all. Both are based on the traditional teacher–pupil relationship.

In our scheme the goal for which we are aiming is rather different. While it is often loosely said that we are trying to train general practitioners to carry out psychotherapy, this is in fact not true.

In order to enlarge on this point, let us compare our course with the only recognized training course in psychotherapy – training in psycho-analysis. Psycho-analytic training is carried on in a unique context in which the candidate learns to understand both his own problems and those of his patients as part of a specific professional training with permission to practise (diploma) as a psycho-analyst as his declared goal. It is hoped, moreover, that the candidate's personality will change and that he will come to have more insight into his personal and social relationships. The ordinary training for psycho-analysis is structured by a highly organized selection procedure, a training scheme with control analyses leading to a diploma granted by the training institution, with agreement between analyst and candidate about the eventual termination of the training analysis, and therefore a formal ending.

In our training scheme, however, there is no such structure. Balint, as the pioneer, felt when he started that he knew so little about the skills involved in the general practitioner-patient relationship that he was unwilling to commit himself or the doctors involved to any formal statement of aims. When the training method emerged from the original seminar, neither Enid nor Michael Balint had any knowledge of the amount of work or time which would be needed to arrive at a degree of understanding and skill that would be generally acceptable. Moreover, they were not even sure whether generally acceptable criteria for the transmission and use of these skills could be found. Therefore the seminars led by the Balints were generally concerned with the doctor's role and with understanding the doctor–patient relationship. This does not in itself call for either the formal structure or the profound personal changes demanded by psycho-analytic training. The aim has been stated succinctly by Balint as 'a limited though considerable change in personality'.

We can say, therefore, that traditional training schemes are either orientated towards time and achievement or, in the case of postgraduate refresher courses, that the whole question of what is transmitted is completely ignored. The training method devised by Balint, however, while setting no time limit for granting a diploma and offering little in the way of lectures or theory, differs in that the emphasis is on the acquisition of psychological skills through the medium of the seminar. Measurement of the achievement of this aim is confused because of the necessary importation into the training situation of the therapeutic paradigm. Moreover, this is an area about which very little is known, and one in which there has been very little research, because of the

17

complexity of the processes involved and the lack of clearly stated criteria.

A further complication has been the attitude of the major institution under whose auspices the Training Scheme has been carried out. Sutherland, in his appendix to *The Doctor, His Patient and The Illness* (Balint, 1957a), states that it is proper for the specialist consultant to devote a proportion of his time to training and *maintaining* a number of general practitioners in their work with psychological problems so that in this way he may make a more effective contribution to psychotherapy on a scale appropriate to community needs. The importance of this maintenance role is that it is, at any rate theoretically, an interminable relationship and thus the maintenance component may be life-long if both parties so wish. The effect of this attitude has been to postpone consideration of the actual effectiveness of the Scheme and to suggest that as long as a certain number of practitioners were occupied in seminars, then the institution was adequately carrying out its role in the community. This idea has added yet another pressure against assessing the work of the Scheme.

Fortunately, the consultants who joined Balint, while accepting the principles involved, have not all taken up the maintenance role to which the institution offered to commit them. Many of them have been fascinated by the possibilities and scope of the seminar method, both for the acquisition of psychological skills and for research into various types of relationship. Certainly, we have always provided one long-term maintenance seminar, which was sufficient for those doctors who became dependent failures, but generally the emphasis has been more on investigation of the possibilities of our method rather than merely providing long-term support for general practitioners.

Structural Aspects of the Tavistock Training Scheme

2. A SOCIOLOGICAL MODEL

When I joined the team in 1961, to assist in the research project into the efficiency of the Mutual Selection Interview, I suggested that without an understanding of the sociological development and structure of the course it would not be possible to evaluate our work and, in particular, the effect of the Mutual Selection Interview. I was struck by the difficulty in relating the effects of selection to the aims and assessments of the course. In order to try to chart the development of the course and clarify the influence of the factors which are described above, I suggested that we use as a model the work of our colleagues of the Tavistock Institute of Human Relations on the Glacier Metal Project (Rice, 1953). In this work Rice describes the use of sociological concepts in examining variations in labour turnover in a factory. In his paper Rice showed that labour turnover in a factory had evolved as a distinct social process with a pattern of its own. He used concepts drawn from Open System Theory and Lewin's Field Theory to study the process of recruitment of labour and termination of employment. He suggested that such concepts might be used by other investigators to study turnover of personnel as a distinct process within a particular institution.

Our first step in developing a similar model for our training scheme was to identify the phases of development in such a social system. In order to do this, we charted a frequency distribution showing the number of general practitioners attending the course from November 1952 to November 1964 (see *Figure 1*, p. 8).

In this figure the ordinate shows the number of general practitioners attending the Tavistock course during any one term; the abscissa shows time from 1952 to 1964.

For each year a count of doctors attending was made at

19

the mid-points of the three terms, and the mean calculated. Examination of this graph suggests that three phases can be described in the development of the Scheme. In each case the phase is defined by a change in the slope of the graph. Historically speaking, these phases coincide with changes in the institutional structure of the Scheme.

Phase 1

The relative flatness of the curve defines Phase 1, which lasted from the beginning of the course in 1950 until 1954. During this period all doctors who applied were accepted, and the teaching method was gradually developed by Balint. During this phase some 60 per cent. of general practitioners attending the Scheme dropped out, as did two psychiatrists who had originally agreed to lead seminars. The population drawn upon was very varied and consisted of experimentally inclined doctors of a very wide range of ages and interests. The average number of practitioners attending during this time varied between ten and fifteen. In 1953 and 1954 Michael Balint and the 'Old Guard' were engaged in working out the technique for training practitioners. Balint kept the group absolutely stable with no members leaving and none joining. Balint also decided not to start any new seminars until this work had been finished. Thus it was Balint's deliberate policy that this seminar should remain completely isolated during this period.

Phase 2

Because of the positive slope of the next part of the curve we have called it Phase 2. Phase 2 lasted from 1954 to 1958 and was one of considerable expansion of numbers. The Tavistock Clinic gave greater support to the course. Balint closed his original seminar and began three new seminars. A second generation of new leaders sat in on these seminars and then began to lead seminars of their own. The implicit decision was made at this moment that seminar leaders needed an in-service training and this could only take place by the method of attending as participant observers and then being allowed to make their own mistakes in their own way as leaders of new seminars. The Scheme began to be more widely known and the total number of practitioners attending at any one time rose to between seventy and ninety. The population of practitioners attending at this time seemed to consist of doctors from more established general practices rather than the more experimentally inclined group of the first phase. During Phase 2, the Scheme itself generally changed its character. From being self-contained, small, and research orientated, it evolved into a postgraduate training event offered by the Clinic to general practitioners and was advertised as such in our training booklet. The relationship between the new leaders and new practitioners was centred on training and was much less research centred than the relationship between Balint and the members of his pioneer seminar. Balint himself became more interested in the extension of his technique of handling seminars, while the new leaders entering the training role brought with them their own interests and problems and a lesser degree of personal identification with the work.

At the same time the organization of the Scheme began to change considerably. The institutional aim was now stated as the training and maintenance of general practitioners using the method devised by Balint. The new leaders entering the Scheme found different roles for themselves. Some began leading new seminars, while one provided a maintenance seminar on the model suggested by Sutherland. Finally, a selection system was proposed as a result of Balint's recognition of the difficulties attendant upon accepting all practitioners who applied to the course.

A Study of Doctors

Implicit in these decisions was the establishment of a scheme with conditions for entry, a common form of training, but no process for disengagement. Each member of the staff had different aims and the difficulties imposed by this situation were underlined by the fact that no time limit was set for training and it was deliberately decided that no agreed method of ending the seminar should be imposed. It was left to the individual practitioner to continue or not, as he wished, though in practice when the number of doctors attending a seminar fell below four, the seminar was terminated. However, all doctors who wished to continue were offered places in other seminars. This process was called 'reshuffle' and it is discussed in greater detail below. It is noteworthy that the practitioners themselves made various attempts both to gain recognition for the course as a postgraduate activity and to gain recognition from the College of General Practitioners and Postgraduate Medical Federation, with a diploma as the eventual goal. On the other hand the Clinic preferred to institutionalize the lack of a diploma and ignored the questions involved in the length of training and the lack of provisions for disengagement. This difference in emphasis has persisted throughout the life of the Scheme.

Phase 3

Once again the curve flattened out after 1958 and this defines Phase 3 which has lasted until the present time. By 1958 the expansion had reached its limits and the demand for places and the number of seminars had more or less reached stability. From that time until 1964 the total number of doctors engaged in the course remained stable at about seventy with some twenty new doctors joining each year and about twenty others disengaging themselves in one way or another. On the staff side the Scheme continued to change since a new generation of leaders joined the staff while Balint reduced his teaching role considerably in view of his retirement from the National Health Service in 1961. The number of psychiatrists participating as seminar leaders remained constant at about seven. Responsibility for the course was taken over by Gosling and the second generation of leaders took on second and third seminars. Contact was made with workers in this country and abroad and a whole series of participant observers, associates and foreign visitors, have attended seminars and contributed to the work both in informal discussions and in the technical seminars which were established after 1961 (see Chapter 1, p. 10). In open system terms, the system had reached a 'steady state' of dynamic equilibrium. To quote Rice: 'If an institution is to preserve its own unique institutional characteristics, its own particular "atmosphere", some form of process is implied which will maintain these characteristics. Such a process is like a river which continuously changes its elements, even if its velocity and direction remain the same.' In particular, such a process has the properties of a self-regulating mechanism. It will show resistance to change, and if disturbed in any way, will show a tendency to re-establish a 'steady state'. This steady state has continued despite Balint's retirement from the Tavistock Clinic in 1961, and the gradually increasing effect of the technical discussions for seminar leaders. On the staff side this phase has been marked by the gradual development and discussion of new modes of thinking about both the doctor–patient relationship and the transmission of skills in the seminar. Demands to theorize about the activities of the Scheme were made both by seminar leaders and by associates. When the writer joined the staff as consultant psychologist, it became possible to undertake the present appraisal of selection. This in turn has stimulated further work and thought about the social processes in the Scheme. At the time of writing (1964) at least three attempts are being made by

23

various members of the staff to undertake research into the training process using different but related sets of hypotheses. One group is studying the relationship between the leader and the seminar; another, possible methods of recording the actual processes involved; and the third, dynamics of the seminar's first year. Other contributions have been made by colleagues abroad. This work has been studied at a series of international conferences.

The model that we have presented is similar in many ways to that described by our colleagues in factories and other institutions. It seems likely that training schemes of the Tavistock type, given sufficient institutional framework and flow of personnel through the system, will tend to develop towards a 'steady state', resist change, and, if disturbed, will strive to re-establish their equilibrium.

3. THE USE OF THE MODEL

By describing the Scheme in this way and, in particular, its arrival at a 'steady state', we have been able to discover how it was that the criteria concerning the success or failure of the course remained undeveloped until we undertook this study. It is, of course, for other schemes to investigate whether this model holds true for their work. For our part, we wish now to examine the processes within the Tavistock Scheme which have contributed to this situation. These may be thought of as the outcome of the interactions of two sets of factors: those which initiated change in the system, and those which resisted it. Among the factors that resist change in the system we have already noted the importation into a Training Scheme of attitudes belonging to the therapeutic situation. These attitudes are part of the admirable medical practice that the therapist is available for as long as he is needed by the patient. However, without any explicit agreement about

24

the end of training, the tendency of the doctor is to cling to the system in the hope of winning through to an idealized solution or to abandon the system without acknowledgement and without a full realization of the disappointment associated in the ending of any meaningful relationship.

A second factor that has protected the system from change has been the lack of study of the doctors' stated reasons for leaving it. Just as the conditions of attachment had been allowed to develop without interference until 1956, the problem of whether the doctor chose either a settled connection on the basis of idealization, dependence, identification, or continued learning, or chose to leave, has been allowed to lie fallow until sufficient material is at hand. This has had the effect of protecting the system, and particularly the leader's picture of his role, and of avoiding the necessity of making any considerable change in the structure of the Scheme.

A third factor militating against change was the introduction of what we called the 'reshuffle'. This first came into operation in 1956 when several seminars became so small that it was impracticable for them to continue. These seminars were amalgamated, and a leader who was new to at least some of the members then took over. This procedure proved useful, and from then on it was applied systematically to all groups of more than two years standing. On these occasions an attempt was made as far as numbers allowed, to put doctors who had shown roughly the same rate of development in their previous seminars together in the new seminar. Thus the faster developers were now surrounded by people of similar ability, as were the slow developers. It was thought that a greater uniformity in the standard of work being done would help the seminar to be both more interesting and more profitable for its members. At the same time one leader undertook a maintenance seminar for all the very long-term doctors. This last seminar was designed to support doctors indefinitely – it was never reshuffled.

These decisions meant that on the whole the system opted for continuity. If doctors wished to continue, they could do so, and facilities were made available to them. We noted in fact that the reshuffle was used by quite a number of doctors as a welcome opportunity to leave. From our point of view it was hoped that the reshuffle would ameliorate conditions of work so that a much more even standard would become possible and the seminars would become more productive. These hypotheses were never examined critically and the reshuffle system has continued very much on a pragmatic basis. We have not been able to confirm that fewer doctors got hurt or left because the level was too high or too low for them. It is also possible that a considerable percentage of doctors disliked the change and left much sooner than they might otherwise have done. Moreover, any attempt to study the effect of the reshuffle was unfortunately hindered from our point of view by two factors. One difficulty was that certain doctors could not come on various days and therefore could not be placed in the seminars that we considered to be appropriate for them; the second difficulty was that various leaders, while reluctantly accepting this system, asked for, and got, one or two favourite, pleasant, or particularly able doctors in their new seminars to compensate them for accepting difficult and disruptive doctors. As a result, it seems that in using this method, seminars that were otherwise quite well matched broke up, and promising doctors were lost. Moreover, it is worth underlining that the implication that, perhaps, a doctor who was stuck might get on better with another leader, has led to a lack of a more vigorous effort to work out and undertake new training techniques.

Among the factors making for change in this system were the introduction of new leaders and the Mutual Selection

Interview. First, new leaders: although one might assume that new leaders going into the Scheme would slip easily into the work after six months or so as participant observers, this did not prove to be so in practice. Thus, despite sharing the psychiatric and psycho-analytic frame of reference, each new leader approached the work with hesitation and with some anxiety. The seminar situation is always difficult for new leaders. This is inevitable, and we feel that the only possible form of training is an 'in-service' training in view of the difficulties and anxieties of the inexperienced seminar leader, whose developing ideas may influence the goals of the system. The different ways of dealing with the anxieties arising in our work in a seminar has resulted in the established techniques being challenged and extended. A forum was set up for this purpose to discuss techniques of leading seminars and other vital topics for seminar leaders. This led in its turn to a series of international conferences at which our techniques were compared with those in use in other countries (see Chapter 1, p. 10).

The second major factor making for change was the introduction of the Mutual Selection Interview. This had the effect of considerably decreasing the proportion of doctors accepted for the course; at the same time, when it was introduced, we had no idea of its efficiency. We believed that it had significantly improved our results. Moreover, we hoped that the number of doctors for whom the Scheme turned out to be a painful and unprofitable experience would have been significantly decreased. However, it was not possible to validate these hypotheses because we had not yet succeeded in describing our vague idea of a better general practitioner, which was the accepted aim of the Scheme.

Among the other factors making for change in the system, which we will briefly mention here, first, the gradual development of a different attitude towards training among some of

the leaders, best exemplified in the work of Gosling and Turquet (1965); secondly, the influx of new generations of
associates and leaders with new ideas which were freely expressed in the technical discussions; thirdly, our continued
contact with colleagues running similar schemes in other
institutions and other countries. One example of this was the
adoption by a number of the seminars of the 'random case
technique'. Balint had suggested studying unselected cases
in the seminar, and the idea was enthusiastically taken up by
groups both here and abroad. An account of this work has
been given by Mitscherlich from Heidelberg (personal communication), where each doctor in turn was asked to present
the tenth case on a specified day in his surgery, thus enabling
the seminar to obtain a picture, not only of the treatment of
cases selected by the doctor, but also a random sample of the
doctor's performance with his patients. Another account of
a similar investigation is soon to be given by E. Balint and
others.

4. SUMMARY

We have used socio-psychological concepts to construct a
model of the General Practitioner Training Scheme. We
have described how the Scheme grew naturally with a deliberate lack of definition concerning conditions of entry,
length of training, and disengagement. We have also described how these conditions became institutionalized and
preserved factors tending towards stability in the operation of
the Scheme. Against these we could put a series of factors
directed towards change and perhaps towards improvement
in the system. It almost seems as if those factors in the
Scheme that arose accidentally were based on unconscious
motives and were conducive to constancy, whereas those
factors that were planned were based on conscious motivation
28

and have contributed to change in the system. Where these were matters of deliberate policy, such as the introduction of the Mutual Selection Interview and the introduction and training of new leaders, it was obviously important to try to evaluate their effect. At present, when the Scheme is considered as a whole, we cannot accurately predict how changes in one aspect of the system will affect the other parts. But we would naturally expect, for example, that a change in conditions for leaving would have repercussions throughout the Scheme, or that a new reshuffle system would considerably change the length of attendance of particular doctors. Unfortunately, at present we do not have the material available to answer these questions fully.

In the remainder of this book we attempt to examine the effect of two of the major factors making for change. We have concentrated our attention on selection and on the introduction of new leaders, since these are variables that can be relatively easily defined and that seem to us to be extremely important for our work. In order to do this, we have, of course, had not only to look critically at the Scheme but also to develop criteria with which to try to estimate the acquisition of skill in the seminars. We have therefore developed a rating scale based on our observation of the doctor's behaviour in the seminar of which he is a member, and our inferences from this behaviour in terms of his treatment of his patients. We have used this rating scale to try to measure the effects both of selection and of the introduction of the new leader; it is with this study that the remainder of the book is concerned.

CHAPTER 3

The Need for Selection
by Michael Balint

---

1. THE PROBLEM

As mentioned in Chapter 1 (p. 4), the first course of seminars for general practitioners was organized at the Tavistock Clinic in the autumn of 1950. To start with I accepted, without any further examination, the generally held belief that every general practitioner, provided he intended to remain in general practice, was a promising and most welcome entrant for any postgraduate or refresher course. It is perhaps worth noting that all over the world every organization or authority which has arranged postgraduate courses for general practitioners has always acted upon this same, unexamined principle, namely, that any refresher course given by a bona fide specialist is suitable for any general practitioner. Since these courses have been as a rule, short-term – lasting at most a week or a fortnight – no one has been compelled to examine in earnest what his results were, and therefore this principle, or belief, has remained unchallenged.

Since my seminars lasted for a considerable time – a minimum of several terms of weekly meetings – a number of problems were quickly encountered. I realized then that if I wanted to find answers to some of them, a long study would be needed. I therefore arranged that a register be kept for every seminar showing the date of its inception, the names of the doctors participating, their attendances and absences, and ending with the date of its winding up. Similarly, each doctor had a card on which we recorded the date of his joining the Training Scheme, each seminar of which he became a member, and the date when he ultimately left the Scheme. At the time of his leaving I added a brief description of my impressions of him, especially of the way he responded to the new experiences and of the presumed reasons for his leaving. Still later, when the Mutual Selection Interview was introduced, that is from 1956, each doctor's card recorded first a brief description of the results of that interview. All these records have, of course, been treated as confidential material.

Both the seminar registers and the doctors' personal cards were continued by my successor, Gosling, and these two instruments form the basis of the present study. In recent years Gosling has introduced a third important source of information – a discussion with each doctor who decides to leave the Training Scheme about his motives for doing so and his impressions of the aims and the success or failure of the course. In the last few months a start has been made by our team, both at the Tavistock Clinic and at University College Hospital, in devising a form for a still more informative recording of the Mutual Selection Interview.

2. EARLY LEAVERS OR SELECTION

One of my first discoveries was that a very great number – more than half of the entrants – dropped out before the end of their first year of attendance at the seminars. This was a real novelty because, as far as I know, no report on

31

postgraduate or refresher courses for general practitioners has ever mentioned anything similar to this. Our finding was the more surprising when it is realized that all our entrants were volunteers who came attracted by our advertisement in the medical press offering discussions of 'Psychological Problems in General Practice'.

I could comfort myself with the knowledge that among those who respond to any offer of a new method, there is always a large proportion of unstable people whose dissatisfaction with the old ways originate not so much from objective criticism as from subjective conflicts. This comfortable assumption – as a comparison of our figures relating to the earlier and to the later years of our Training Scheme will show (see Chapter 6) – was partially correct, and could explain some part of my early findings. Of course, it could have been argued also that probably the same phenomenon occurred in every postgraduate course organized for general practitioners. The difference between my seminars and the other courses was that the others did not, and could not, know that this was happening because of their short duration, which did not allow sufficient time for this development to become apparent.

But, whatever the reason, a decision had to be made. Should our training method be changed to suit a greater number of volunteers, or should some arrangements be made to select the suitable ones, or – still better – to enable the applicants to get to know something about the seminar method so that, if they found it uncongenial, they could withdraw before having committed themselves?

Evidently this was to be an important decision which would profoundly influence the future of our Training Scheme. As described in Chapter 1, the final form of our training method was worked out with the help of the 'Old Guard' in the years 1953-4 and tested out with two more

32

The Need for Selection
groups of doctors during 1955. By that time, as will be described in more detail in Chapters 4 and 6, I had collected enough data about the doctors who had dropped out early from the course to be able to formulate some ideas of the reasons for their leaving. On this basis – apart from a general principle to be discussed below – several groups of early leavers were isolated with fairly sharp diagnostic characteristics, e.g. the seriously neurotic, the 'superior', and the obsessionally conscientious. All these will be described in detail in Chapter 4. A close study of these early leavers led me to the decision not to alter either the aims or methods of the course, but to introduce a selection procedure, which will be described in Section 3 of this chapter. At that time, in 1956, I am sure I could not have formulated the exact rationale of my decision; I only felt that we must preserve certain standards. Here I shall try to state more precisely what I then had vaguely in mind.

The nature of any training scheme is determined by four interrelated factors:

1. its aims,
2. its methods and techniques,
3. the quality of its staff,
4. the quality of its entrants.

The interrelation between these four factors is so close that if any three of them are held fairly constant, the fourth can move only within very narrow limits.[1]

The aim of our Scheme right from the start has been, first, to develop in the doctors a sensitivity to their patients' emotional problems, to enable them to understand these

[1] Factors 1 and 2, our aims and methods, will be described by Enid Balint and myself in a separate book, which is in preparation under the title *Training for Psychotherapy*. Here I shall deal with these two factors only very briefly and shall have to refer the reader to the coming publication.

problems more safely and at a greater depth, and then to help them to acquire skills in using this understanding for the goal 'of therapeutic effect. A precondition for the acquisition of this increased sensitivity and therapeutic skill is a general loosening up of the doctor's personality, especially with regard to his professional work. He must be able to notice and to tolerate emotional factors active in his patients that he rejected or ignored before, and he must learn to accept them as worthy of his attention. I have called this total process as '*limited though considerable change of his personality*'[1] (Balint, 1957a).

The essence of our training method, that is factor 2, has been:

(*a*) to expose the doctor to the full weight of his therapeutic responsibility, not allowing him any tacitly accepted escape;

(*b*) to contrast his individual ways of treating his patients with those of his colleagues in the seminar;

(*c*) to use the group setting to demonstrate that any form of therapy entails a specific type of interaction between patient and doctor, the nature of which can be understood and the future development of which – and with it the efficacy of the therapy – can often be predicted.

Incidentally, this specific nature of our training method is the explanation of one of my earliest discoveries, that without the pressure of constant and on-going therapeutic responsibility, our method proved, as a rule, unsuccessful.

---

[1] This does not mean that the aim of the course has been to change general practitioners – or, for that matter, specialists – into psychiatrists; but rather to enable them to become better general practitioners or specialists. Admittedly, in a few cases, in fact in less than 2 per cent. of all our entrants, the doctors have decided to change over to psychiatry. This outcome was assessed as a relative failure of our Scheme and certainly not as an unqualified success.

Furthermore, this responsibility had to be active at the time
when the doctor attended the seminar, and neither memories
of past, or prospects of future responsibilities could be
substituted for it. To give two examples: we admitted on
occasions doctors who, after several years in general practice, had accepted appointments in the public health service,
and missionary doctors who wanted to use their customary
long leaves to learn something useful for their future work;
all of them proved to be either failures, or only limited
successes. Apparently the pressure of actual and constant
therapeutic responsibility is an essential factor for our
sort of training. Remarkably, the same was true for a few
specialists who insisted on joining a general practitioners'
group. The reason for the only limited success achieved
in their case seemed to lie in the nature of their different
type of contact with their patients. A specialist sees his
patients for a limited period and for a limited aim, while
a general practitioner's contact with his patient is fairly
general and has hardly any limitations in time. I stated
this important finding regarding the limitation of our
method as follows: *the seminar method can train doctors
for the work that they are doing at present, but not for work
that they have done in the past or expect to do in the future.*

Evidently this training method, which is based on making
vague or even repressed experiences fully conscious in the
doctor, on enabling him to accept and tolerate them instead
of turning away from them, and – what is still more difficult
– to work with them in a detached, professional manner,
requires a leader who is familiar with the unconscious and
its mechanisms. This means that, if at all possible, the staff
must be recruited from trained psycho-analysts or, at least,
from dynamically oriented psychiatrists – our factor 3.
We know of a number of attempts in this country at dispens-
ing with this restriction; as far as we know, none of them

can be called successful. The same is true, on the whole, for similar attempts in the United States. The only exceptions to this rule are in Holland, but we feel that the undeniable success achieved in that country has had to be paid for by a somewhat lower standard than seems acceptable to us.

In our Training Scheme, colleagues who joined it as leaders at its later stages accepted my decision about standards. As an experiment, therefore, factors 1, 2, and 3 have been kept fairly constant during the almost fifteen years of our existence. Admittedly there have been a few inevitable variations which have had their repercussions in the groups of doctors affected by them. The connections between these variations and their effects will be dealt with partly in Chapters 6 and 7 and partly in the coming publication. Since these variations were only limited, we may take it, for the purpose of this chapter, that the aims and methods of training, as well as the quality of the staff engaged, were kept fairly constant.

Since three out of the four factors have intentionally been kept constant throughout the existence of the Training Scheme, the fourth factor, the nature of the entrants, could move only within rather narrow limits; in other words, only a certain sector of the general medical population have been able to benefit from what has been offered to them.

3. THE MUTUAL SELECTION INTERVIEW

The decision taken in the mid-nineteen-fifties, that the original aims of our Training Scheme should be preserved and the methods worked out in the research period be continued, meant that we had to accept the fact that some doctors would not be able to make use of our method of training. So I was faced with the obligation of working out a selection procedure. I had to cope here with two sorts of difficulty: one objective, the other subjective.

As described, by 1956 I had some ideas about what types of doctors made up our early leavers, our most conspicuous failures. These, however, were vague and only qualitative; they gave me no indication as to how much of any given characteristic should be considered as giving a bad prognosis, how much could be passed as negligible, and how much as an acceptable risk. In addition there was the then fairly large group of 'one-term doctors' which, as described in Chapter 4, meant in fact that I was proved incapable of making a diagnosis on them for the time being. All this suggested to me that I should be free with my hunches, but very cautious with my judgements.

The other difficulty was purely subjective. I hated the idea of examining colleagues who had expressed interest in my ideas and volunteered for my seminars, and of then telling them in an authoritative way that they were found unsuitable. I felt this humiliating for them as well as distasteful for myself.

The solution for both sorts of difficulty was found in a type of interview which might be called a Mutual Selection Interview. In general, when one speaks of selection, one has in mind a procedure that would enable an employer to choose from among the applicants the most suitable person for a particular job. In this procedure, the employer is the authority who actively selects, while the applicants are the material that passively permits itself to be chosen or otherwise. In contrast to this general idea, the interview, as we conduct it, is a mutual selection, an interaction between two more or less equal partners.

Usually, when a doctor applies for a course of instruction, he has a fair idea of what he is getting into from the published details of the course and from analagous experiences he has already had, for example, at university or school. Our training course, however, is unlike anything he is likely to have met before in that it directs his attention as much on to his own personality and idiosyncrasies as it does upon the traditional object for study in medicine, the patient. Indeed, at times it upsets the whole basis of his medical training, which is to emphasize the difference between the ill patient and the healthy doctor, and instead casts the two together as the object for study. In any selection procedure for our Training Scheme, this novel feature needs to be brought to the applicant's attention in some way more convincing than a mere verbal statement of fact.

In the first years of our Scheme, doctors were confronted with this novel approach only after they had joined a seminar, and it was only then that they were able to decide whether in fact this was something they wanted to have and with which they could or could not work. Similarly, the leader could assess only from his experience in the seminar whether the seminar's ability to work profitably was enhanced or obstructed by the way any particular doctor was behaving, according to the dictates of his personality.

The aim of our selection procedure has therefore been to remove some of this trial period from the course itself and to confine it to an event occurring before the seminar began, i.e. the selection interview. This meant two things: first, that the selection must be a mutual selection, and second, that it was the job of the interviewer, among other things, to give the applicant a sample of what he might expect if he joined a seminar, so that he might have a chance of rejecting the course if he found the sample uncongenial.

Obviously an interview between two people cannot be the same as a seminar of a dozen or so different, and as yet unknown, people. Nevertheless, the interviewer, by refusing to do all the interviewing himself and by encouraging the applicant to notice and to consider this fact and its results, gives the applicant a taste of what it is like to be in a seminar that is more concerned with fits and misfits between people than with anatomy and physiology. Although quite early on in the interview either the applicant or the interviewer may have provisionally made up his mind to accept or to reject the other, it is the interviewer's task to try to bring to light more evidence against which to test this provisional decision.

I usually start by explaining that our respective expectations must be compatible, or else our collaboration may prove difficult, or disappointing, and that the aim of the interview is in fact to find out how far our expectations are mutually compatible. For the next step the point is not so much whether the doctor starts by talking about his expectations, or I about what the seminar would expect from him; rather, the important thing is that he is shown a sample of what is likely to happen in the seminar, the interviewer representing the aims of the course as well as the possible behaviour of the seminar, including its leader.

It is the interviewer's task to do this in a manner that will enable the doctor to react to this presentation in his own individual way. This in turn will enable the interviewer to attempt to recognize, diagnose, and classify the doctor's individual reaction and, if necessary, reinforce it by his own responses in an appropriate way. While still under the influence of this fairly intense experience, the doctor is asked to review his initial decision to apply for the course, taking especially into account whether or not, in his view, the mutual expectations will be compatible.

This whole interaction between applicant and interviewer, if properly conducted and observed, provides ample material for the assessment of the doctor's potentialities in the seminars, of which the atmosphere and ways of working are well

39

known to the interviewer. It is worth mentioning that in the overwhelming majority of cases, the two decisions have been identical. This may sound remarkable, but it is only a natural consequence of our whole attitude and the atmosphere in which this interview is conducted.

This procedure has been used in well over 200 cases, mainly by Gosling and myself, and an open clash of opinions has occurred only six times. The pattern then has always been the same; the doctor has begged us to accept him, but we have felt unable to do so; this happened exclusively in cases diagnosed by us as severely neurotic or 'superior' doctors. Apart from these overt clashes, there have been some more covert ones: I am referring to those doctors who agreed with the interviewer to come to the course but withdrew before it could start, or failed to respond to our letter informing them of the date on which the new seminar was to start. It is likely that a large number of these doctors belong to one special group – C_5 – which will be described in Chapter 4 and which we intend to study in the future. We are aware of the existence of another type of group about which it is well-nigh impossible to obtain reliable data: I refer to those doctors who, perceiving that the interviewer does not intend to accept them, agree with him in order to avoid an argument. This group too should be studied, but we do not know yet how this may be done.

When re-reading our records of the early Mutual Selection Interviews for the purpose of this research, we discovered to our dismay that our descriptions were not detailed nor our predictions precise enough. In order to remedy these shortcomings, we recently devised a form for recording our initial findings and predictions. This form is at present undergoing constant modification. When working on this chapter, I realized that the new form ought to contain the following observations: (*a*) the doctor's initial expectations of the course, (b) how these changed under the impact of the interview situation, and (c) his final decision and his reasons for arriving at it.

4. SUMMARY

The title of this chapter is 'The Need for Selection'. What I want to show is that if we accept our aims as worthwhile and our methods as sensible, we must accept also that only a proportion of general practitioners will be able to benefit from our Training Scheme. We developed a selection procedure – the Mutual Selection Interview – to enable some doctors to withdraw without too much disappointment and bitterness and before they had committed themselves too deeply. Our figures, to be discussed in Chapter 6, will show to what extent this selection procedure has proved its worth.

This, however, is only one part of the question. The other part asks: is this restriction acceptable? Would it not have been much better if we had revised our uncompromising aims, reduced them to more practical levels, and, *pari passu*, developed less exacting methods that would then have made this highly important field accessible to a larger proportion of general practitioners? This is a question of fundamental importance, but I must ask the reader to wait until Chapter 8 in which we discuss it in detail. But before we reach that stage, we have several other tasks.

Until now we have discussed only our obvious failures, that is to say, the doctors who had to leave the seminars too early, before they had had enough time for the acquisition of the necessary therapeutic skills. Does this mean that every doctor who stayed longer than, say, a minimum of one year can be considered a success? We have never had any thought in our minds that this might be so. Staying for a sufficient time is a necessary condition for learning something, but it is certainly not enough. In order to assess the efficiency of our training, we have had to develop a scale for rating the doctor's sensitivity in understanding his patient's problems and his therapeutic skills as they have developed during his connection with our Scheme. This rating scale will be discussed in the next chapter.

CHAPTER 4

Principles of Assessment *by* Enid Balint

---

1. AIMS AND BASIS OF CLASSIFICATION

The system of classification to be presented in this chapter is the result of an historical development that proceeded almost unnoticed. Our system therefore has very little theoretical foundation; it is based on our growing clinical experience. Its two main aims are: (*a*) to evaluate the efficiency of the Mutual Selection Interview described in the previous chapter, and (*b*) to enable us to study the results of our Training Scheme.

The first variable of our rating system is simple, straightforward, and unequivocal. It is the length of time before the doctor decides to leave the Scheme. This is a continuous variable which we divided into the following classes:

Class I: doctors leaving during their first year.
Class II: doctors leaving during their second year.
Class III: doctors leaving during their third year.
Class IV: doctors leaving after more than three years.

We had to introduce two additional classes: 'Transfer', doctors who left us to change over to another similar training scheme, and 'Still Attending', which means that on the census day the doctor had not yet left the Scheme.

Our second variable represents an attempt to integrate

43

responses to two different problems that appeared at two different periods of our development. The first, which became apparent in 1955-6, was that a sizeable proportion of our doctors left too early – the obvious failures of our Scheme; it was thought that if their reasons for leaving were properly understood, both the disappointments and the waste of energy and time could be avoided. Attempting to solve this problem, Michael Balint studied the group of early leavers, i.e. the doctors who left before the end of the first year, and described them in 1957. On the basis of this work, and with the aim of reducing their number, the Mutual Selection Interview described in the previous chapter was developed.

Our first task, then, when undertaking this research was to extend and systematize his work so that all those doctors who left early could be described in terms of their apparent reasons for leaving. This principle of classification is mainly a diagnosis of the doctor's motives for leaving. I shall return to this important point later in Section 5.

The second problem we had to face became apparent only after we had started the study on which this book is based. Michael Balint always realized that in itself the fact that a doctor stayed in the Scheme did not mean that he was a success. He accepted this as self-evident and did not attempt to measure the various rates of progress or the ultimate level that each individual doctor reached. When, however, we were faced with the task of validating our selection procedure, we had to ask ourselves whether the fact that this or that doctor stayed for several years in our Scheme was to be considered as success or failure or, more correctly, in what proportion or from what angle it should be considered failure or success. This led to an extension of the original system of classification which initially covered only the early leavers.

For the classification of this group, which we call the late leavers and stayers, we use another principle which might be called the study of the interaction between the group and the doctor. This will be described in Section 3.

We wish to stress that although our system of classification appears continuous – and perhaps there is even some element of continuity in it – we are fully aware that it originated from two different sources and that the effects of these two origins are unmistakably present. At the end of this chapter, I shall discuss the uncertain transitional area that resulted from our attempt at integrating the two scales.

Before going any further, I would point out that all the material used for this rating consisted of phenomena of a tripartite interaction between one particular doctor, one particular group, and one particular leader; as a rule this was then simplified by neglecting the influence of the two other factors and attributing everything observed to the particular doctor. This seems justifiable, but only as a first approach, since the influence of the other two factors, though present, is more constant (see Chapter 7, Section 2 and Chapter 8, Section 4). Indeed, in grading doctors according to their ability to use the seminar, we are grading the leaders' ability to help doctors to achieve this aim and, ultimately, we are rating our whole method of training. These connections on the basis of statistical material will be discussed in Chapter 6.

This, then, is the main reason why our rating scale does not intend to – in fact cannot – say anything about the doctor as a general practitioner. What it tries to assess is the doctor's interaction with our Scheme. In fact we know from outside sources that a number of doctors who were among our very early leavers, and thus must be considered as failures, are in fact excellent general practitioners. This is an important point that must be borne in mind all the time when reading this book. What, therefore, we describe as failures are, in fact, failures of our Scheme to help a particular doctor to acquire the skills that he asked from us.

2. THE EARLY LEAVERS

As mentioned in the previous chapter, one of the earliest discoveries of our Training Scheme was that only doctors who are under the actual and continuing pressure of therapeutic responsibility for their patients can be trained by our methods. In consequence we omitted from our study all doctors who either were not general practitioners at all or were not engaged in general practice at the time when they attended the seminars. In any case, most of these belonged to the early phases of our history because later, when we learned from our mistakes, these doctors were not accepted.

The first category in our classification comprises those doctors whose reason for leaving is external to our training and is, perhaps, prior to it. We called this Class A and divided it into two sub-classes. A_1 comprises doctors who for some reason or other could only attend the course for a limited period. Quite often the external reasons for the limitation of time were compelling and convincing, but their effect inevitably was, in most cases, to enable the doctor to remain uninvolved in his patients' problems, as well as in those presented by his colleagues; thus his experience in the seminars did not make the necessary impact on him.

Sub-class A_2 was called 'insufficient intelligence'. Although a medical qualification may, perhaps, be considered as an adequate intelligence test, some people get through it who apparently are unable to mobilize enough intelligence to follow the intricacies of the seminar discussions. To our surprise there were a few failures for whom this appeared to be the only acceptable explanation.

The next category, Class B, contains all our diagnostic failures: it comprises the doctors who stayed so short a time, or left so weak an impression behind them that we were unable to diagnose sufficiently the reasons for their early departure. To cover our failure we call them – following Michael Balint

46

who first described them – 'one-term' or 'nondescript' doctors. We must repeat that this means only that we know very little about them. We are glad to observe that with improvement of our Mutual Selection Interview and of our diagnostic ability, the number of Class B doctors constantly diminishes.

The last group of early leavers, Class C, contains all the doctors whom we could describe in diagnostic terms. This is a large and important class, divided at present into four subclasses, three of which were described by Michael Balint in 1957. The fourth was added during the present research. It is possible that we shall have soon to add a fifth, but this sub-class is not yet clearly defined.

Some volunteers to our courses – Sub-class C_1 – were found to be suffering from serious neurosis, or even borderline psychosis and possibly were attracted to the course in the hope of getting therapy in an indirect way. Some of them were persuaded to seek therapy openly; others dropped out when they realized that their unformulated or indirect expectations would not be met; last, a few had to be asked to discontinue their attendance – a very unwelcome task for the leader and one seldom resorted to.

Another group of early leavers – Sub-class C_2 – was made up of what Michael Balint described as 'superior' doctors. These were well established, experienced, and successful practitioners with excellent reputations both among their patients and in the profession, who had a very strong 'apostolic fervour' which was almost certainly a defence against insecurity. From the outset they tried to teach their own methods and were practically incapable of listening to, still less seriously considering, any methods other than their own. This inevitably brought them into competition with the psychiatrist/leader who represented the aims of the seminars, and this resulted in a strained and tense atmosphere. After some unsuccessful attempts to convert the rest of the seminar to their 'faith', these doctors dropped out, dissatisfied and critical.

A third group of early leavers – Sub-class C_3 – was made up of conscientious and sensitive practitioners. Their practices and their patients meant a great deal to them and they seemed a promising group, apparently more than willing to learn. Moreover, they remained with us for two or three terms, or even a little longer, and left us reluctantly, apparently struggling with a conflict. They were designated by Michael Balint 'obsessionally conscientious characters', and we took over his description. What they repeatedly asked for, and apparently needed, were reliable rules, efficient time-saving methods, intellectual problems which could be discussed and solved with detachment and objectivity and, above all, no personal psychological involvement. Our unstructured and deliberately unpremeditated ways made no sense to them. Possibly they did not wish to expose themselves to the 'considerable, though limited change of personality' which, as discussed in Chapter 3, is the prerequisite of our Training Scheme.

Sub-class C_4 was isolated during our present research. This group comprises doctors who are fully aware that their methods need improving and even that they themselves need to change. They feel insecure and wish to change, but because of some form of neurotic anxiety, this change appears to them too frightening. This conflict remains for some time unresolved but then something, apparently entirely unconnected with their personalities, unexpectedly happens in their external circumstances, and, regretfully they have to leave.

There are a few early leavers who do not fit into any of these four classes. We have seen so few of them that we do not yet know whether they should be constituted as a separate class – C_5. Their main characteristic is that they appear to have good and successful defences. Their emotional life is

48

acceptable to them; their professional successes are good; and, in the first approach, they appear to be well adjusted and fairly normal people. However, the Mutual Selection Interview reveals several topics which they prefer to avoid. They feel the interview itself a considerable strain and at the end of it are glad to be offered an opportunity to withdraw or to postpone their decision. Although in every other respect they seem to be most promising entrants, we felt, at any rate for the time being, that their wish to withdraw should be respected and not challenged (see Chapter 6, p. 83).

This sub-class was recognized in the Mutual Selection Interview and is described here mainly for future reference because we think that some of the B or even D_2 doctors might fall into it.

3. LATE LEAVERS AND STAYERS

In Section 1 we referred to some of our difficulties in deciding on what factors to base our assessment or rating of this group. It could have been something external to our seminars, that is, something additional to and independent of them; on the other hand the basis could have been the doctors' behaviour in the seminars. Each of these solutions had its advantages and disadvantages. After some deliberation we decided for the second alternative, that is, to use only what we ourselves could observe in the seminar setting. To state it more precisely, we base our rating solely on the ways the doctors reported their own cases and took part in the discussion of those of other doctors. This classification, therefore, is based on assessing the changes that took place in their capacity as participants in the seminars, changes which were brought about by their attendance.

Before devising this part of our scale, yet another question of principle had to be decided: what kind of standards should be used. Should the standards be absolute, expressed in terms of what we would expect from every doctor? Or should they be relative, expressed in terms of what could be expected from each individual doctor according to his own potentialities? After much consideration, we decided to use the absolute standard and to make no allowance for individual idiosyncrasies or weaknesses.

The advantage of our method of classification was that we did not interfere with our doctors by visiting them and we made no intrusion into their private or professional lives. It is true that this limited our horizon, but in basing our evaluation on the ordinary happenings in the seminar, we avoided any extraneous elements that might have confused our relationship with the doctors. In contrast, at the Staunton Clinic in Pittsburgh, a large-scale research is being carried out in which a team of observers visits each doctor four times a year in his surgery, and a classification is thus based on observing his professional work. Because of lack of funds this method was beyond our capacity; but in any case it would have been somewhat alien to our way of thinking.

Our method of rating clearly had disadvantages too. Since we did not see any doctors individually after the selection interviews, and were never directly in touch with their work as general practitioners, and since they were not obliged to report their experiences in their practices to us unless they felt inclined to do so, it might seem that we must often have been at a loss to know in which category to place them. It is always difficult to know in our field what has been achieved through the training. In addition to the above limitations we have no examinations; our doctors are not at any time expected to answer questions or write papers. Nor can the ways in which a general practitioner treats mentally ill people be used as a basis for assessment because this is only a very minor part of his daily work. It is, therefore, largely irrelevant whether the doctor has greater or less successes with his mentally ill patients.

In spite of all these disadvantages no leader found it too difficult to assess the doctors in his seminar. True, his contact with them was limited, but this contact in the seminar was intense, continuous, on-going, and of long enough duration to enable the leader to build up a sufficient knowledge of each individual doctor for his assessment.

It must be added that though the classification of any one doctor is the expression of what one particular leader thought of him after having observed him for some time in his seminars, the structure of our Scheme has been such that every doctor who has stayed for any length of time – that is all our stayers or late leavers – has automatically been a member of several different seminars and has therefore been observed by more than one leader and reacted to more than one group of doctors. We will discuss in Chapter 5 to what extent various leaders agreed and disagreed about the category in which each doctor should be placed.

First, we divided the group of late leavers and stayers, purely on a phenomenological basis, into two sub-groups: the one comprising the doctors in whom we could not observe any, or only minimal, changes during their period of attendance at the seminars; the second group was made up of those doctors in whom substantial changes were observed.

At first we thought that the class showing minimal or no change, Class D, was nothing but a sort of protuberance of the Class C, especially the Sub-classes C_2, C_3, and C_4. The only difference, so we thought, was that the Class D doctors somehow or other managed to stay longer and thus escaped being categorized as C. In fact we even tried to act upon this idea and to classify the Class D doctors, using similar principles to those we found useful in classifying the C doctors. This attempt failed.

51

Some of us went even further and thought that in a way it was a mistake that we have kept our Class D doctors so long; rightly they ought to have been allowed, or even encouraged, to drop out earlier, like the Cs. In this way, perhaps, they would have been spared a good deal of useless effort, perhaps also some irritation and disillusionment, and our hard-pressed Scheme would have gained some valuable time.

It was not easy to dispel the persuasive power of these ideas. This was the more difficult because to some extent they were correct. This discovery – that our preconceived ideas were true for some of the Class D doctors but were untrue for others – came early in our present research; but it only increased our confusion. It was only after a detailed study of groups B, C, and D that we realized that our confusion was caused by our own failure, in as much as we had not separated clearly in our mind the three different principles of rating that we had used automatically.

The first principle is phenomenological, and this was adopted as the basis of our rating system. The second, which is inseparable from any analytical thinking, is dynamic; it asks what are the mechanisms of the minimal or no-change reactions and what are their significance for the doctor. The third principle is a value judgement; although there is only minimal change in the doctor's behaviour in the seminars, has he, or have his patients, gained anything from his experiences in the seminar?

It was on the basis of these considerations that we finally decided to sub-divide the D class into two sub-classes, D_1 and D_2.

In our experience the doctors belonging to Sub-class D_1 are, as a rule, some of our most regular attenders. They fall into two groups. They are either almost silent participants, hardly ever reporting cases; but in spite of this they are certainly not withdrawn, and they appear to follow the discussions with interest. It is rather difficult to form an opinion as to why they attend the course since on the rare occasions on which these silent doctors decide to speak, they give the impression of not 'going along' with the developments of the seminar, either in its ideas or in its spirit; apparently they do not even try out new ways of behaving to, or thinking about, their patients. Often what they report seems strangely inappropriate.

In contrast with them, the other group of doctors belonging to Sub-class D_1 are unusually lively and active. They appear willing, even enthusiastic, to try out new solutions to their problems; their performance, however, seems to prove that they have not really grasped the problems with which the group was grappling. Perhaps there is never real sympathy or harmony between them and the group, and thus the influence of their new experience does not result in a purposefully orientated change in their treatment of their patients; similarly they themselves become no more at ease or relaxed in their work.

The doctors belonging to Sub-class D_2 are, on the whole, neither silent nor over-active. From time to time they report cases and take an average share in the discussions. Their comments, though not usually outstanding, are more or less to the point, and in due course they show some slight, but not very great, change in their handling of their patients' problems. They are pleasant members of the seminars who create no disturbances. Although it is clear that they have gained some general understanding about the importance of the doctor–patient relationship, this is rather patchy and unreliable; moreover they find some difficulty in using it in a purposeful way and are not entirely confident as to its relevance in their work. In contrast to the doctors belonging to Sub-class D_1, however, they become increasingly relaxed with their patients and more at home with their colleagues in the seminars.

B   53

In our opinion the dividing line between success and failure runs through Sub-class D_1. We are convinced that some of the doctors belonging there should definitely be considered failures, whereas others – with some optimism – might be classified as qualified successes. We feel that almost all the doctors belonging to Sub-class D_2 are clear successes. Our impression is that not only have they themselves gained a lot, but also that they are able to carry this gain over to their practices and give a better and more understanding service to their patients.

The same is true, but to a much greater degree, for our next two classes. Here there can be no doubt that their attendance at the seminars has brought about the 'limited though considerable change of personality' that we consider a necessary prerequisite for the acquisition of therapeutic skills in human understanding.

The first of these, Class E, is defined as 'definite changes but of uncertain quality'. These doctors have not only learned to understand in a general way the importance of their interaction with patients for the better understanding of their patients' problems, but they can also use this knowledge purposefully for therapy. As a rule they are active and useful members of the seminar; they are quite sensitive to what is going on in other doctors' cases in the doctor–patient relationship and can use this to make relevant comments; they are not afraid of reporting their own cases even when these reports show them in an unfavourable light. They are open to new insights and can make use of them when meeting their patients next time. However, their use may on occasion tend to be clumsy or ill-timed, apparently because they are more impressed by what the leader said or by what happened during the seminar discussion than by what the patient is trying to tell them in the here-and-now situation in their surgeries; in this way they often are one step behind the patient. A great number of them give the early impression that they can and will continue to change; in fact they make quite a commendable progress for a year or so; then they lose momentum and can apparently go no further. This, however, is true only of some, not of all.

Last, we have Class F, which consists of doctors who made a positive change of a substantial and reliable quality. Not only have these doctors gained in understanding, but they have also acquired reliable skill in using it purposefully. Of course, like everybody else, they are liable to make mistakes, but this they can accept. Moreover it quite often happens that when reporting a case they themselves notice where they have missed a point or blundered. They can also accept criticism of their blind spots and stupidities and equally are helpful in their comments on the case reports of their colleagues. One may add that in the few cases in which we could follow these doctors after they had left the seminars, we had the impression that, in contrast with the doctors belonging to Class E, changes continued in them, and they continued to develop. On the other hand, with doctors in this group who were still attending the seminars, we sometimes had the impression that they appeared, like the doctors in Class E, to have reached the limit of possible change and then suddenly and unexpectedly they showed unmistakable signs of deeper insight or of new, more reliable, or more sensitive skills. This is a most interesting observation which is well worth further examination.

4. THE RATING SCALE

We include here our complete rating scale with the instructions. These, of course, are much shorter than our descriptions in Sections 2 and 3. They aim to help the psychiatrist/leader in making his assessment as much in line with those of his colleagues as possible.

GENERAL PRACTITIONER CLASSIFICATION

MARK VIII   DECEMBER 1963

General Remarks: This classification takes into account evidence of changes in three facets of the doctor's behaviour: (1) in his manner of presenting cases; (2) in his participation in the discussion; and (3) in his reported handling of cases. All the classes refer to interaction between the doctor and the seminar except for Class A which refers only to the doctor's resources. Wherever possible, sub-classification should be used, e.g. C_3. Terms in parentheses refer to Balint's original classification in *The Doctor, His Patient and The Illness* (1957, pp. 315–20).

Early Leavers (roughly up to one year)

A. Limitation[1] of:
   1. Time.
   2. Intelligence.

B. Reason for leaving is quite obscure: doctor is nondescript and does not disclose himself, or he discloses himself but leaves unaccountably (one-term doctor).[2]

C. No change and
   1. Very severe neurosis or borderline mental condition (seriously neurotic doctor).
   2. Rigid character defences which, when threatened, lead to disruptive or supercilious behaviour (superior doctor).
   3. Insecurity with obsessional defences: he leaves disillusioned on discovering that he cannot get simple and reliable rules (obsessional doctor).
   4. Insecurity with neurotic anxiety; change is desired but is too frightening; external circumstances are

---

[1] This class refers to the doctor's resources only.

[2] This class acknowledges our failure to be able to draw inferences about the doctor–seminar relationship.

often used as an excuse for leaving. He is an *over-anxious doctor*.

Late Leavers and Stayers (more than one year). They can tolerate the seminar.

D. Minimal changes
  1. His behaviour in the seminar and his reported hand-ling of patients indicates little or no change.
  2. His behaviour in the seminar indicates increased understanding of the cases discussed, and some liber-ating of knowledge which perhaps he already had but which was unavailable to him previously. In his cases this slight increase in understanding is shown rather in feeling more at ease with his patients and in toleration to them than in his deliberately apply-ing it when considering what to do.

E. Definite changes but of uncertain quality.
  He can usually contribute to and learn from the seminar; what he learns he applies in his practice and the result is brought back to the seminar for further work. He becomes more flexible in the seminar and more versatile with his patients. As his understanding of his cases increases he develops new skills in handling them which he applies consciously and deliberately. His understanding, however, while accurate, may lack immediate relevance; experience in the seminar appears to weigh heavier than experience with the patient; he appears to copy others rather than to respond in a new way of his own.

F. Definite changes of substantial quality.
  As for E, but in addition his understanding comes to include a sense of what is relevant in his ideas and observation; his remarks therefore are more appropri-ate and meaningful. He can learn more from the patient

57

than from the seminar and can notice some of his mistakes and can then recover from them.

5. COMMENTS

In concluding this chapter, I should like to make some general comments.

First, I wish to repeat what was said in Section 1, namely, that all the observations upon which the ratings have been based have the structure of a tripartite interaction between one individual doctor, the group of doctors of which he is a member, and one particular seminar leader. For Classes D_1 to F we infer from these observations the ways in which the individual doctor relates to his patients: whereas for Classes A–C what is inferred is the doctor's reasons for leaving. That is why we have little idea as to what happened between a doctor and his patient in Classes A–C, and what reasons the doctors had for leaving in Classes D–F.

In addition this is the explanation as to why there is a much stronger correlation between our rating and the length of stay of the doctors in our Scheme than we think is justified. All these shortcomings might disappear if we had a unified rating scale based only on one principle; but we have unfortunately not been able to develop one. As an inadequate substitute for this unified scale we propose in the future to study the doctors belonging to the transitional area between the two parts of our present rating scale.

It is also worth repeating that in rating the A doctors we say nothing unequivocal about suitability of the doctor for the course, or of the course for the doctor. In rating the C doctors, however, we are led by the doctor's behaviour in the group which forces him to leave. This rating does not say anything about the doctor's relationship with his patients or whether he is a good doctor or not. What it does say is some-

58

thing about the neurotic interaction with the leader and the members of the seminar.

Doctors belonging to Classes D, E, and F are rated as such because they are able to stay in the Scheme. They are differentiated further according to their way of reporting their own cases and participating in the discussions following other doctors' reports.

A doctor is classified as B because he leaves too early to enable the seminar leader to have enough time to understand him.

It is important to bear in mind that not all these classes are clear cut and precise. They are sharply delineated in some directions, but their contours are rather vague in others, as it ought to be in this kind of classification since these decisions depend not on a qualitative but on a quantitative judgement. For instance, it is easy to see that it is at times difficult to decide whether to place a doctor in Class C_1 or C_2. In other cases similar difficulty might arise between Class C_1 and C_4. In fact, C_4 might be considered as a central group from which gradual steps may lead, on the one hand, towards B and C_1 or, in the other direction, towards D.

Finally, one might say that the doctors belonging to Classes C_1, C_2, and D_1 are those doctors who are problems to the leaders and possibly also to their colleagues in the seminars; whereas the doctors belonging to Classes C_3, C_4, and D_2 are the doctors who may have problems within themselves.

CHAPTER 5

Use of the Rating Scale
by Robert Gosling

WHEN we came to apply the rating scale to our population of doctors, we had first to find out how reliable it was in the hands of those who knew the doctors well, namely, the seminar leaders.

Accordingly, at one of our regular staff meetings we asked our colleagues, who had already been given a copy of the rating scale, to criticize it and discuss its use. The discussion highlighted two defects. The first was the difficulty introduced in the middle of the scale by the change in the kind of inference to be made; though all inferences were to be based on observation of the doctor's behaviour in his particular seminar, in the first part of the scale they were to be concerned with his reasons for leaving it, while in the second part with the way he related himself to his patients (see Chapter 4). This change proved very hard to grasp, and then to operate. The second defect highlighted was the ambiguity as to whether, when doctors were still attending a seminar, the rating was to be on his present performance or on his apparent potential for development; for example, of two doctors showing about the same capacity for understanding their patients and for using this understanding in their treatment, one might give the impression that he would always follow slavishly the lines taken in the seminar, while another might show promise of becoming more independent and self-reliant. The discussion also indicated a good deal of unwillingness to be saddled with so onerous a task and some suspicion as to whether the validity of the results would make the effort required worth while.

In the light of the discussion, and of the effort needed later to get the rating scale actually applied by our colleagues, we divided them into three categories; first, those who had taken an active part in devising the scale and who were heavily committed to using it effectively, namely, the authors of this book; second, those who were thinking along similar lines but were less emotionally involved in the research; and third, those who had little sympathy either for the approach or for the task, or for both. Even so, it should be emphasized that all those applying the scale came from a fairly uniform background: in addition to being qualified psycho-analysts they also shared an interest in applying their experience in psycho-analysis to work done in groups, whether groups for therapy or for training. They had also had numerous opportunities in the past few years to discuss together their efforts in leading seminars for general practitioners, and so had developed something of a common language.

1. RELIABILITY

Our first task was to determine how consistently a seminar leader applied the scale to the same doctor on two occasions, the two occasions being far enough apart to minimize the effects of memory. Two of the authors rated doctors who had worked in their seminars and had already left either early or late; fourteen months later they were asked to rate the same doctors again retrospectively without being told their previous ratings. They were inconsistent with their earlier ratings three times out of thirty, one leader once and the other twice. The inconsistencies were F to E, E to D_2, and D_2 to D_1.

For the purpose of this research the critical point in the scale comes between classes D_1 and D_2, since doctors rated from A to D_1 are considered failures of our training while above this point they are considered successes. As classes A to C are defined unequivocally by their leaving the Scheme early, little inconsistency is to be expected in the application of that part of the scale. Most interest lies therefore in the efficacy of the scale in differentiating the D_1 class from those higher, distinguishing failure from success, and then in differentiating the higher classes from each other, i.e. D_2, E, and F, distinguishing degrees of success.

When rating the same doctors twice our two authors classified four doctors as D_1 on the first occasion and five on the second, i.e. one inconsistency in five. As expected, none of the inconsistencies occurred at the A to C end of the scale, to which ten doctors had been assigned; they all occurred at the D^1 to F end, i.e. three inconsistencies out of twenty.

It was only after this first test of the scale's reliability had been made that we realized that only the second half of the scale needed to be examined, i.e. D_1 to F. Not only is this half of the scale the one that calls for finer judgement when the scale is being used, but also it refers to issues that are central to such a training scheme i.e. the ways in which a new professional skill is acquired and manifested. Moreover, for administrative reasons it was easier to collect a fair number of ratings for comparison if attention was confined to those doctors who had stayed longer than one year. From this point on, therefore, our examination of the rating scale's reliability was confined to that of its second half only, the four classes D_1, D_2, E, and F.

We then asked two colleagues in our second category –

i.e. those interested but not so much involved – to rate again doctors whom they had rated previously at the time of their leaving more than ten months before. As all the doctors concerned had stayed longer than a year, only the second half of the scale was applicable. They were inconsistent with themselves three times out of twenty-one comparisons, one seminar leader once, F to E, and the other twice, D_2 to E both times. The D_1 class was assigned five times and occasioned no inconsistencies.

In our third category of colleague – i.e. those not much interested in the rating scale – inconsistencies were much more frequent, e.g. six times out of fourteen comparisons; the D_1 class was assigned seven times, three times inconsistently.

Thus, seminar leaders who were considerably or moderately committed to the task of applying the rating scale were consistent with themselves thirty-five times out of forty-one comparisons (85 per cent.) when applying that part of the scale calling for considerable judgement and consisting of four classes (D_1, D_2, E, and F). In the use of the critical class, D_1, they were consistent with themselves nine times out of ten. On no occasion were they inconsistent by more than one class.

We then turned to the question of how far there was agreement between different psychiatrists. As the first category of colleagues, the authors of this book, had compared notes so much already, it was thought meaningless to measure the amount of agreement between them: what independence in rating there might have been had got lost in their efforts to find an agreed way of expressing their experience with doctors they had all known. It is presumed that they were closely consistent with each other in their use of the scale; this presumption was not, however, tested.

To get two simultaneous and independent ratings on the same doctors, we had to turn to seminars that included, beside the leader, a participant observer who had attended long enough to become familiar with the ways in which the various doctors worked. The seminar leaders who took part in this experiment were of one or other of our first two categories. The participant observers, though interested enough to undertake the rating and to have attended a seminar consistently, were nevertheless not all equally committed to the Training Scheme nor familiar with the ideas lying behind it. Despite this, they consented to rate the doctors without previous discussion of the procedure and without any special training in it.

In two of the pairs that rated doctors simultaneously the participant observers were closely identified with the aims and method of the Scheme, and indeed had themselves at times acted as seminar leaders. One pair agreed nine times and disagreed three times (E and F, E and D_2, E and D_2) and the other agreed five times and disagreed three times (E and D_2, E and D_2, D_2 and D_1). In another pair the participant observer was one of the authors of this book and so was very familiar with, and committed to, the training technique. He agreed with the seminar leader four times and disagreed with him an equal number of times (D_1 and D_2, D_1 and D_2, D_2 and E, D_2 and E). It will be seen that these disagreements were all in the same direction and appear to reflect a difference in the stringency with which the scale was applied. In the fourth pair the participant observer had identified himself so little with the work that he had not taken part in any of the technical seminars for the staff and had indicated in various ways that in addition to being critical, he was even hostile to much that was going on. He agreed with the seminar leader six times and disagreed five times (D_2 and E, D_2 and E, D_2 and E, D_2 and D_1, F and D_2). As can be seen, these disagreements are not all in the same direction, and in one case disagreement is by more than one class.

Taking these four pairs as a representative sample of the psychiatrists who may use the rating scale, we can expect agreement between them 62 per cent. of the time (twenty-four times out of thirty-nine comparisons). On only one occasion was the disagreement greater than by one class, i.e. 7 per cent. of disagreement. (With the same distribution of disagreements among the four classes, a difference of more than one class would be expected 40 per cent. of the time if chance alone operated.) Moreover on no occasion was a doctor rated by one psychiatrist as D_1 but put higher than D_2 by the other. Agreement between psychiatrists rose to 97 per cent. if it was taken to mean that either the same or an adjacent class was assigned by the pair.

The rating of such complex variables is always difficult and the reliability of such scales is never very high. For comparison we may point to the well established and clinically useful field of x-ray diagnosis. In describing the extent of pulmonary tubercular lesions shown on chest x-rays, according to the widely used three point-scale of the National Tuberculosis Association, experienced observers were consistent with themselves in 83 per cent. of cases and agreed with each other in between 50 and 70 per cent. of comparisons. When assessing such x-rays for evidence of activity of the disease on a three-point scale observers were consistent with themselves in 71 per cent. of cases and agreed with each other in 50 per cent. of comparisons; if only differences greater than one class were counted as errors, these figures were increased to 93 per cent. and 77 per cent. respectively (Newell, Chamberlain, and Rigler, 1954). Similarly, if the course of the disease was rated on a three-point scale, using serial chest x-rays, observers were consistent with themselves in 97 per cent. of cases and agreed with each other in 70 per cent. of cases respectively (Yerushalmy, 1953).

As x-ray diagnosis has been found to be a useful tool in

the clinical management of pulmonary tuberculosis, its reliability, as given above, may provide us with a point of reference. When using our rating scale, observers were consistent with themselves in 85 per cent. of cases and agreed with each other in 62 per cent.; if only differences greater than one class were counted as errors, then these figures were increased to 100 per cent. and 97 per cent. respectively. From this we conclude that as a clinical instrument the rating scale is fairly reliable. In the following chapters the rating performed by the leader of the last seminar attended by the doctor was invariably the one used for providing the statistical data.

When we then came to use this imperfect tool to rate changes in doctors over the course of time, it is hardly surprising that the results obtained were inconclusive. In reviewing our records we found that the same doctor had worked with different leaders for periods of a year or more on seventy-nine occasions: thirty-two doctors were rated twice, sixteen on three occasions and five on four occasions. The later leader gave the same rating as the earlier one fifty-one times; fourteen times he rated him higher, and the same number of times he rated him lower. On only two occasions did their ratings differ by more than one class. Thus six times out of ten the comparisons indicated that there had been no change. No overall pattern could be detected when these comparisons were scrutinized, but some interesting points deriving from them will be discussed in Section 2.

As all these ratings were done after the doctor had completed at least one year of his training, nothing can be said of changes appearing during his early days (see Chapter 8, Section 3). Evidently our scale is not sensitive enough to trace changes in the later years of training. The amount of agreement between the ratings of successive seminar leaders seemed to indicate either that what changes there were had taken place during the first year, or that by and large it was the doctor's potential for development that was being recognized and rated and not his present level of attainment. It could also be that our Training Scheme produced no changes of any importance in the doctors attending it; but this possibility is opposed by the widely held opinion that at least some of those attending developed quite considerable new skills.

2. SOURCES OF ERROR

When our colleagues met together to discuss our difficulties in demonstrating changes in degree of skill with this rating scale, five points emerged.

First, it was evidently very hard for some colleagues to resist rating doctors according to their apparent potential for development; this prognostic slant seemed to them to be essential. Although the scale, as it existed, referred only to present behaviour, it may be that such a formulation precludes some useful and possibly invaluable information that can come from the psychiatrist's clinical sensitivity. Almost identical behaviour on the part of two doctors may yet in its accents and nuances betray to the experienced observer the difference between a man who habitually hangs back and a man who, though cautious, may be on the threshold of personal innovation. Though psychiatrists' opinions in these matters are notoriously inconsistent with each other's, it would be ludicrous at this stage to sacrifice seminal ideas for the sake of reproducibility.

Second, despite overt acquiescence in the thinking behind the rating scale, different psychiatrists evidently used it differently according to the slightly different aims they consciously held for their trainees. Although these differences were mainly of emphasis, they often led to discrepancies in rating. The most obvious difference was between those who hoped the seminars would enable the participants ultimately to engage upon some kind of dyadic, face-to-face, verbal psychotherapy, and those who expected the understanding gained to be used by the family doctor in a variety of ways, many of which might be quite foreign to the practice of the psychiatrist/leader. Occasionally this difference in emphasis led one leader to rate a doctor highly and another to express his disappointment by giving a much lower rating.

The third point to emerge was the unconscious aberration of judgement that all leaders suffered at times; despite the incredulity of his colleagues, a leader would persist in an opinion about a doctor's performance and express it in such a way as to indicate to the others that he had a 'blind spot' for this man. Sometimes he would seem to some extent to be enchanted by a particular doctor, and sometimes to be dealing with his *bête noir*.

In addition to influencing the leader's rating, the intrusion of unconscious factors undoubtedly played an important part in the working of the seminars, and so in their results. For reasons that might remain obscure to all concerned, a doctor sometimes found one leader far more compatible than another and so able to facilitate his development to a greater extent. The same could be said of the psychiatrist's own sense of compatibility with different doctors. This 'counter-transference' component to the leader's approach, therefore, influenced the doctor's actual behaviour in the seminar on which the rating was based in addition to the way the leader perceived him.

The fourth point was also one referring to the leader's own personality, namely, his tendency habitually to overrate or underrate all doctors with whom he worked compared with his colleagues. Although each series was too small to produce reliable figures, there were indications that, in their first seminar, leaders tended to underrate their doctors compared with what their colleagues saw of them later; there were also indications that those leaders with a strongly therapeutic emphasis in their training aims tended to over-rate their doctors as if they had been stimulated by signs of mental health to take an over optimistic view of what was being achieved in training.

The fifth and final point was the interesting fact that while some doctors seemed always to require the same rating whether by the same leader on successive occasions or by different leaders, others were always extremely difficult to classify. It was as if some had a fairly uniform level of per-formance and an unambigious way of communicating it to any leader, while others were either very variable in the skill they could master at any given moment or they presented themselves in the seminar in such a way as to leave the leader always in doubt about them. These two extreme types were identified only late in this research and so their significance is not yet known.

In summary, therefore, we may say that in the hands of the majority of our colleagues the rating scale gives fairly reliable results in identifying our so-called successes and failures. In about 90 per cent. of cases leaders gave the same rating when asked to rate the same doctor repeatedly. When the same doctor was rated by two different observers simul-taneously but independently, the ratings were identical in about 60 per cent. of cases. If an adjacent class as well as the same class was allowed when assessing agreement between a pair of observers, this figure was increased to about 95 per cent. The scale is not discriminative enough to trace changes in the doctors' skill in the later stages of training. Difficulties in using the scale consistently can be accounted for by (*a*) the presence of complexities and ambiguities in the structure of the scale, and (*b*) variable performance of doctors and variable rating by seminar leaders due to the intrusion of different conscious aims and unconscious prejudices on the part of the leaders.

CHAPTER 6

Evaluation of the Selection Procedure
by Peter Hildebrand

---

1. THE TAVISTOCK POPULATION AS RATED ON THE SCALE

In the previous chapters we have described our rating scale and the principles on which it has been based. In this chapter I shall examine the changes in the distribution of doctors among the various classes of the scale and describe the changes brought about in our population by the introduction of the Mutual Selection Interview.

The Mutual Selection Interview was introduced in 1956 – so the doctors attending our seminars fall naturally into two groups. One group comprises all doctors who entered the Scheme without any selection procedure in the years 1950–6. We have called this group of doctors the Pre-selection Series. The other group entered the Scheme after the introduction of selection interviews in 1956, and we have divided it into two sub-groups. The first sub-group, which we have called Post-selection Series I, comprises all the doctors who entered between Easter 1956 and 31 July 1960. This was the series we originally planned to compare with the Pre-selection Series. However, because of the length of time taken by the planning and carrying out of this research, we were able also

70

to include a second sub-group, called Post-selection Series II, which comprises those doctors entering between 1 August 1960 and 31 January 1963. All the doctors were rated either at the time when they left the Training Scheme or, if they were still attending, by the leader of the seminar in which they were participating in January 1964, i.e. by the person who had the most immediate contact with them.[1]

Thus even the most recent recruit in Post-selection Series II had had at least four terms' experience in a seminar at the time he was rated. We were able to differentiate between the early leavers on the one hand, and the late leavers and stayers on the other (see Chapter 4). For the purposes of this chapter, I have called those doctors who fall into the ratings $A-D_1$ i.e. all early leavers, plus those doctors who stay but learn nothing, 'failures', and those doctors who are rated D_2, E, or F 'successes'.

Table 1 below shows the distribution of the seventy-two doctors in the Pre-selection Series according to their length of stay (see Chapter 4, p. 43) and the final rating given to them by the seminar leaders (see Chapter 4, pp. 46–55). For ease of comparison the table gives not only absolute figures but also percentages. The reader will see that in addition to the ratings which will be familiar to him from the earlier chapters, there are five doctors rated X. These doctors were members of a seminar which was terminated prematurely by the leader after two terms. We have therefore kept them separate from the other members of the series, and we regard them as failures of our Scheme.

---

[1] Many of those doctors who came in the early years of the Scheme of course left before we had constructed the rating scale. However, Michael Balint had always insisted on writing full notes about the performance of all doctors who joined; these notes were used together with discussions with the leader of the last seminar which the doctor had attended to arrive, where necessary, at a retrospective rating.

TABLE 1. RATINGS OF ALL DOCTORS IN THE PRE-SELECTION SERIES

	X	A	B	C_1	C_2	C_3	C_4	D_1	D_2	E	F	Total	%
Class I	5	8	13	6	3	4						39	55
Class II					1		1	3	2	1		8	11
Class III								3		1		4	6
Class IV									2	3	4	9	12
Still attending								4	2	2	1	9	12
Transfer								1		1	1	3	4
Total	5	8	13	6	4	4	1	11	6	8	6	72	100
Sub-totals	5	8			28			11		20			
%	7	11			39			15		28			

In *Table 2* we have set out for comparison the ratings for the doctors in Post-selection Series I. The total number of doctors in this group is 109. One doctor in this series was originally a member of the seminar that was terminated prematurely; he returned to the course and later transferred to a parallel training scheme at the Cassel Hospital. He was rated X and treated separately from the other doctors in this series.

Table 3 gives the ratings for the forty-two doctors in Post-selection Series II. For ease of comparison we have given separate percentages in each of the three tables for the early leavers rating B–C$_4$, the late leavers rating D$_1$, and the late leavers rating D$_2$–F ('successes').

We knew that the comparison between the various series was made more difficult by the high proportion of doctors attending for a limited time (missionaries, foreign visitors, and the like) in the early days of the Scheme. Secondly, as noted above, one seminar had been terminated by its leader after only two terms. We therefore extracted both the limited-stay doctors, rated A, and the doctors rated X, from each series and then compared the two refined samples in terms of the rating scale. We found that only 33 per cent. of the Pre-selection Series were rated as D$_2$–F ('successes') compared with 66 per cent. rated D$_2$–F in Post-selection Series I. Making the same comparison with Post-selection Series II we found that 63 per cent. of the doctors who joined during this period were rated as D$_2$–F. The difference between the Pre-selection Series and the two Post-selection Series is highly significant. Conversely 39 per cent. of the Pre-selection Series left in their first year of training compared to 20 per cent. after selection interviews had been introduced. This difference again is statistically significant. We consider this to be an important finding since we know that a minimum stay of one year in one of our seminars is a condition without

TABLE 2. RATINGS OF ALL DOCTORS IN POST-SELECTION SERIES I

	X	A	B	C_1	C_2	C_3	C_4	D_1	D_2	E	F	Total	%
Class I		5	2	3	4	2	8		1	4		29	27
Class II		1	2				1	3	3	5	1	16	15
Class III								3	1	5	1	10	9
Class IV								1	6	2	4	13	12
Still attending								6	13	11	4	34	31
Transfer	1							1	2	1	2	7	6
Total	*1*	*6*	*4*	*3*	*4*	*2*	*9*	*14*	*26*	*28*	*12*	*109*	
Sub-totals	1	6			22			14		66			100
%	1	6			20			13		60			

74

TABLE 3. RATINGS OF ALL DOCTORS IN POST-SELECTION SERIES II

	A	B	C₁	C₂	C₃	C₄	D₁	D₂	E	F	Total	%
Class I	2	1	–	1	2	5	–	1	2		12	29
Class II							2	2	8		6	14
Still attending							3	13			24	57
Total	*2*	*1*		*1*	*2*	*5*	*5*	*16*	*10*		*42*	
Sub-totals	2			9			5	26				
%	5			21			12	62				100

75

which it is impossible to acquire the appropriate psychological skills.

On the other hand there are no significant differences at all between the two Post-selection Series; so for the rest of this chapter we have combined them. It may be remarked that there are no ratings of F in the second series. A plausible explanation is that four terms is probably much too short a training period for any doctor to develop far enough to be given an F rating. This point is discussed at length by Michael Balint in Chapter 8. In order to make these comparisons easier for the reader, we have set out in *Table 4* below a condensed version of the preceding tables, expressed in percentages only.

TABLE 4. PERCENTAGE OF SAMPLES
COMPARISON OF RATINGS

	$X \& A$	B	$C_1 \& C_2$	$C_3 \& C_4$	D_1	D_2	E	F	Total
	%	%	%	%	%	%	%	%	%
Pre-selection Series I	18	18	14	7	15	8	12	8	100
Post-selection Series I	7	4	6	10	14	23	25	11	100
Post-selection Series II	5	2	2	17	12	38	24	–	100

Inspection of *Table 4* confirms the important changes that have taken place in the character of our populations. For example, 18 per cent. of the Pre-selection Series were rated B. They were doctors who stayed such a short time or left such a weak impression behind them that we were unable to describe them sufficiently well to give them a C rating. Only 3 per cent. were rated B after the introduction of the Mutual Selection Interview. Clearly on the one hand the selection procedure has served to reveal more of the doctor's personality, his style, and his behaviour and has thus helped us to identify the bad risks of the B rating before they entered the Scheme. On the other hand we have learned to make more precise diagnoses about those doctors who stayed with us for even a short time. The saving involved in reducing the B class, i.e. doctors who did come once or twice to a seminar and then decided that our work was not for them and withdrew, is very evident.

In the present C rating, which comprises the doctors whom we were able to diagnose, the change is also very marked. In the Pre-selection Series the percentage of doctors rated as C_1 ('seriously neurotic') and C_2 ('superior') was 15 per cent. – more than twice as large as the percentage (6 per cent.) of 'obsessional' and 'over-anxious' doctors in classes C_3 and C_4. In the two Post-selection Series, however, this ratio is reversed with the percentage of C_1 and C_2 dropping to between 2 per cent. and 6 per cent. while the percentage of anxious and insecure doctors increased to between 10 per cent. and 17 per cent. We consider that the C_1 and C_2 doctors are failures of selection, while we accept many C_3 and C_4 doctors as necessary risks and regard their failure as a failure of training. As we know, the Mutual Selection Interview was devised to try to help some of the doctors we thought might prove bad risks – foremost amongst them the 'seriously neurotic' and 'superior' doctors – to recognize that the training experience might be painful, or even a threat to them, and help them to withdraw rather than to involve themselves in what might turn out to be an unhappy situation for all concerned. It seems clear that from our figures the Mutual Selection Interview has succeeded very well in this task.

2. A SELECTION EXPERIMENT

This considerable shift both in the length of time that our general practitioners stayed in the seminar and in the amount of skill they displayed was very satisfactory. We naturally wish to attribute the increase in length of stay and the acquisition of new skills to the introduction of the Mutual Selection Interview. However, prudence suggested that we should consider the possibility that this improvement was partly, or even wholly, due to factors other than selection. My colleagues asked me to try to devise some method of evaluating our selection procedure that would enable us to reject such a possibility. They also wished to know if more could be said about those doctors who decided not to join the course, and if we might be creating a situation in which promising doctors were being excluded by some aspect of our approach. This was a difficult task because it could only be carried out retrospectively in view of the time needed before a judgement could be made about the doctors' success in the Training Scheme. A particular difficulty was that the notes of the Mutual Selection Interviews had not been recorded in a uniform manner or, indeed, with any idea that a subsequent study of selection would be carried out. Nevertheless, as our figures definitely suggest that the Mutual Selection Interview has contributed to increasing the efficiency of the Scheme, we hoped that this evaluation would help at the least to establish new formulations as the basis for future work.

I began by discussing at length with Balint and Gosling the principles on which they based their Mutual Selection Interviews. All the records of interviews between 1956 and 1961 were then given to me for scrutiny. The decision on each applicant was recorded by the interviewer, but I had no information relating to the length of time those doctors who joined the Scheme had remained in a seminar. Nor had I any idea of the quality of their work. As no rating scale was in existence at that time, I had, of course, no idea of their eventual ratings. I therefore decided that as there were considerable variations both in the quality and quantity of the notes, the most constructive approach would be one based on the principles used for interpreting projective tests. Since I was not aware of similar work on this sort of interview, I decided to devise my own categories, although I got a great deal of help from discussions with my colleagues. After considerable hesitation I devised a series of categories that I thought would be correlated with a successful career in the Training Scheme and would also be likely to have been recorded by the interviewer, a psychiatrist. I next read the notes of each interview with care to see if they provided information from which I could infer the presence or absence of these particular categories for each doctor.

In some cases this proved not to be possible because of deficiencies in the records. But I was able to devise eight categories for which there were reasonably frequent data and which I thought would have considerable bearing on the doctor's failure or success in the Training Scheme. Because of the difficulties I have mentioned and the subjective nature of the work, I did not expect a great deal from this experiment and I warned my colleagues that we could claim very little support for our hypothesis because of the scientific weakness of retrospective evidence. As noted above, in no case did I know of the subsequent fate of the doctor.

The eight categories at which I finally arrived are set out below:

1. *'Signs of disturbance'*

    The recorded presence of one of the signs used by Balint in his original account of the selection procedure, i.e.

    S.N. 'seriously neurotic'

Sup. 'superior' doctor
Obs. 'obsessional' doctor
Lack of the sign was not scored.

2. *Ordinary Confusion*

Scored when the recorded interview gave the psychologist the impression that the psychiatrist had seen the doctor as really sure neither of himself nor of the implications of his involvement in a seminar. Presence of this sign suggested a good outcome for the practitioner in the seminar. Lack of this sign was not scored since, as so often in this study, the consultant was not obliged to record it.

3. *Impression of Self*

The interview as reported gave the reader some clear impression of the doctor's personality and ways of dealing with others. Presence of this sign was scored positive; absence was not scored.

4. *Impression of Practice*

Some impressions of the doctor's practice and of his attitude towards it. Presence of this sign was scored positive; absence was not scored.

5. *Awareness*

An impression from the interview that the practitioner was aware of psychiatric needs either in the practice or in himself. Presence of this sign was scored plus. A clear lack of awareness was often reported, and this negative finding in those cases was scored minus.

6. *Communication*

An impression that the communication between the doctor and the psychiatrist had been free and natural was marked plus. The opposite impression was marked minus. Where no clear impression could be gained from the notes, no score was given.

7. *Evasiveness*

Some facet of the doctor's personality that the consultant felt was being consciously concealed during the interview was scored minus. Absence of this sign was not scored.

8. *Prediction*

Where a consultant had made, explicitly or implicitly, a favourable prediction, this was recorded plus. Where the prediction was unfavourable or uncertain, this was recorded minus. No score was given where there was no prediction.

Using these categories, I hoped that I might at least differentiate those doctors for whom the Mutual Selection Interview had been an acceptable introduction to the course from those doctors with whom we agreed that we were not meant to work together. In *Table 5* below I have set out the complete figures for doctors applying to the Tavistock Clinic for training in the period covered by Post-selection Series I.

TABLE 5. TOTAL DOCTORS APPLYING TO
TAVISTOCK CLINIC IN POST-SELECTION
SERIES I

	No. of doctors	
Mutually divergent	45	⎫
Probably divergent	7	⎬ did not join
Apparently convergent	11	⎭
Convergent	70	⎫ Post-selection
Interviewed but no record available	39	⎬ Series I
	172	

Of these 172 doctors, 63 did not join the course and 109 did. We have analysed the interview records below.

Psychiatrist and doctor agreed in eighty-one cases (seventy convergent plus eleven apparently convergent) that the doctor

81

should try the course because there seemed to be enough mutual interest to make this worthwhile for both parties. The term 'convergent' was used to indicate agreement to give the course a try, but as we shall see below, eleven of these doctors, about 12 per cent., changed their minds before they actually attended a seminar.

For forty-five doctors, the Mutual Selection Interview resulted either in a mutual agreement that the course did not represent what the doctor was looking for, or in a request that the doctor should reflect on his reasons for applying to get further experience as a general practitioner, or to read Michael Balint's book *The Doctor, His Patient and The Illness*. Only one of these doctors has made a further approach to the course. The psychiatrist expressed grave doubts about the suitability of most of this group of doctors. From the doctor's point of view it seemed that the Mutual Selection Interview provided a graceful and protected escape route. Moreover, I noted that the psychiatrist considered that thirty-three of these forty-five doctors (i.e. 75 per cent. of the sample) showed signs of disturbance. In terms of the signs used by Balint in his book, twenty-three were felt to be 'seriously neurotic', six were 'superior', and four were 'obsessional'. Both for these doctors and for the psychiatrist the Mutual Selection Interview highlighted the difficulties that would probably complicate their attendance at the course. We called this group of doctors 'divergent' since we felt that both parties accepted that their own ways of working and thinking about general practice lay in such different directions as to make collaboration hardly profitable for either side.

I thought at first that I would compare this group directly with the group of doctors whom we found to have ideas which were reasonably congruent with our own. I was not, however, able to do this immediately because, when I checked on the fate of those doctors who seemed to march together with us at the interview, I discovered that eighteen of those who had been recorded as mutually acceptable never in fact attended seminars. This was a surprising finding because the period under review had been one in which the pressure for training had been at its most intense. I consulted my colleagues about this and asked them to check their recollection of these interviews against the records. We then found that we could divide this group of doctors into two classes. In the first class of seven doctors, the psychiatrist had made an offer of a seminar to the doctor who was therefore marked as 'accepted' for training by the Scheme, but it was nevertheless clear that this acceptance by the psychiatrist was meant much more to save the doctor's face and to give him an opportunity to reject us and to withdraw without too much hurt. These doctors really belong to the 'divergent' group although we have kept them apart. We therefore called them probably divergent for the purposes of analysis.

In the second class, consisting of eleven doctors (about 5 per cent. of the total), both the doctor and the psychiatrist were enthusiastic about future collaboration and the psychiatrist generally predicted that the doctor would have a successful career in the Scheme. We do not know what happened to these doctors. We can only assume that they had second thoughts about us which decided them against coming. We regard this class as failures of diagnosis. However, in 1964, Michael Balint had to interview a number of applicants in the course of this work and tentatively identified a group who behaved in a similar manner; he called them C_5 doctors. This group is discussed in detail in Chapter 4, p. 48, and Chapter 8, p. 125. It seems likely that these enigmatic doctors of ours would fall into the same group.

As noted above, we called the group of doctors with whom we were in agreement that the course might prove a profitable experience for both parties the 'convergent' group. We have interview records for 70 out of 109 of these doctors. We have set out in *Table 6* below the incidence of features relating to my eight categories for each group together with appropriate percentages. The three groups are the 'divergent' doctors, the 'convergent' doctors, and the 'apparently convergent' doctors – those who had second thoughts about coming. There were clearly marked and highly significant differences between the convergent and divergent groups. The divergent groups were judged to show signs of disturbance significantly more often and gave a much less clear picture of themselves and of their practices. The convergent doctors

TABLE 6. COMPARISON BETWEEN DIVERGENT, CONVERGENT, AND APPARENTLY CONVERGENT GROUPS

Total	All Divergent 52		Convergent 70		Apparently Convergent 18	
	No.	%	No.	%	No.	%
Signs of disturbance:						
'seriously neurotic'	25⎫					
'superior'	8⎬37	(71)	16	(23)	4	(36)
'obsessional'	4⎭					
Ordinary confusion	9	(17)	15	(21)	2	(18)
Impression of self	18	(35)	41	(58)	10	(91)
Impression of practice	8	(15)	42	(60)	5	(45)
Awareness of psychiatric needs: self	15	(29)	39	(55)	9	(82)
Awareness of psychiatric needs: practice	7	(13)	10	(14)	4	(36)
Lack of awareness	18	(35)	5	(7)	1	(9)
Communication good	10	(19)	30	(43)	7	(64)
Communication poor	29	(56)	9	(12)	2	(18)
Evasiveness	14	(27)	9	(12)	2	(18)
Prediction: good	6	(12)	41	(58)	9	(82)
poor	10	(19)	14	(20)	0	
none	36	(69)	15	(21)	2	(18)

communicated far more easily with the psychiatrist, who in turn predicted success for them significantly more often than for the divergent doctors.

It might be objected that the absence of any figures for one-third of our doctors makes this comparison invalid. We were, however, able to compare the ratings of the group who had been interviewed but for whom the interview was not recorded with the ratings of the rest of the series. Their ratings are given in *Table 7* below. It will be seen that the percentage of 'successes' is 69 per cent. which exactly parallels the Post-selection Series as a whole. For this reason we think it unlikely that there was any profound difference between the group who were interviewed and for which a record was kept and those who were interviewed but for which no record remained.

TABLE 7. NO SELECTION INTERVIEW RECORDED

	A	*B*	C_1	C_2	C_3	C_4	D_1	D_2	*E*	*F*	*Total*
Number	2	2	1	1	2	–	4	8	12	7	39
%	5	5	3	3	5	–	10	20	31	18	100

It is fair to assume that the Mutual Selection Interview has acted as a successful screen. It has enabled those doctors to opt out whose personality or views made it difficult for them to accept the idea of our Scheme. A considerable majority of these doctors seemed to the psychiatrist who interviewed them to be so disturbed that they would be unsuitable for the course. Naturally this does not reflect on their professional capacities nor on their aptitude to undertake other less demanding types of training. More than that we cannot say as we have had no further contact with them. On the other hand we shall discuss the characteristics of the convergent group in greater detail in Chapter 7.

3. A COMPARISON WITH SIMILAR TRAINING SCHEMES

We were fortunate that a further check on the utility of this selection procedure could be made. In this section we compare our results with those of three similar training schemes. They are those conducted by the Cassel Hospital in Richmond, Surrey; the Sigmund Freud Institute in Frankfurt-am-Main, and the Staunton Clinic of the University of Pittsburgh, Pennsylvania. All three courses follow the Balint model in their training and have rated their doctors on our rating scale in order that we may compare results.

Let us make the comparison with the Pittsburgh training scheme first. From the beginning of the Pittsburgh scheme all applicants have been accepted without an interview, and no attempt has been made to predict the outcome of the doctor's participation in the scheme (Pittenger, personal communication). At our request the seminar leaders in Pittsburgh rated each of their doctors on our scale. The results are set out in *Table 8* below.

TABLE 8. RATINGS OF ALL GENERAL PRACTITIONERS TRAINED AT THE STAUNTON CLINIC

A	B	C_1	C_2	C_3	C_4	D_1	D_2	E	F	Total
4	11	1	5	4	1	8	11	5	2	52
65%						35%				

The parallel between the Pittsburgh group and our Pre-selection Series is striking. The percentage of 'failures' is almost exactly the same as in our Pre-selection Series, with large clusters in Class B (eleven, or 21 per cent.) and Class D_1

(eight, or 15 per cent.). A very high percentage of both samples dropped out in the first year; 65 per cent. at Pittsburgh and 66 per cent. at Tavistock. This supports our thesis that without a Mutual Selection Interview a high proportion of doctors who are attracted by the idea of a training scheme in psychology will understandably find that it is unsuited to their needs, with a consequent unsatisfactory outcome for all concerned.

A second comparison can be made with the Cassel Hospital at Richmond, where the two psychiatrists responsible for the course have had their in-service training in Tavistock seminars and have worked closely with us afterwards. Here applicants have been interviewed and an attempt has been made to predict performance in the seminars. However, no one was turned away and only incomplete records were kept so that the predictions were of limited value. We have been given records for twenty-seven of forty-four doctors in the sample. Fifteen were correctly predicted as potential successes or potential failures. For the remaining twelve the predictions were not correct. Considering this finding the correctness of the prediction seems a matter of chance. Main (personal communication) has informed us that in his view the Cassel Hospital should provide a training service for all the doctors in the region, and that therefore no question of mutual selection was involved. We therefore expected that the pattern of the Cassel Hospital group would conform to that of our Pre-selection Series and the Pittsburgh sample. The ratings of the Cassel Hospital doctors by their seminar leaders are set out in *Table 9* below. The number of early leavers and late leavers who do not change, i.e. 'failures', is twenty-four or fifty-five per cent., which supports our hypothesis.

Finally, we have records from a small seminar run at the Sigmund Freud Institute. There the group of doctors were

TABLE 9. RATINGS OF ALL DOCTORS ATTEND-
ING THE CASSEL HOSPITAL TRAINING COURSE

A	B	C_1	C_2	C_3	C_4	D_1	D_2	E	F	Total
2	6	2	2	6	3	3	7	11	2	44
55%						45%				

carefully interviewed and selected according to the following criteria:

(Loch, personal communication)

1st choice doctor: this meant that the doctor was judged on the basis of the interview to be well suited for the seminar and its aims. The doctor appeared well balanced and predominantly motivated by 'interest', less than by needs of his own.

2nd choice doctor: this meant that the doctor was judged to be a doubtful candidate on the basis of the interview. He displayed signs of intensity, irrational thinking and magical ideas and was unclear as to the aims of psychotherapy.

The ratings for the Frankfurt group by the psychiatrist are set out in *Table 10* below.

TABLE 10. RATING OF ALL DOCTORS
ATTENDING THE FRANKFURT SEMINAR

C_1	C_4	D_2	E	F	Total
1	1	3	3	1	9

Where predictions were made five were correct and two incorrect.

The first doctor to leave had stayed a year and a half, so

that in terms of longevity this seminar seems to have been extremely successful. Unfortunately, we have no information about the doctors who were excluded. Certainly, although the seminar was an isolated experiment and no definite conclusions can be drawn from it, the introduction of a selection procedure seems to have contributed to the excellent result.

In *Table 11* below, we have condensed these results into one table.

TABLE 11

	$A-D_1$		D_2-F	
	No.	%	*No.*	%
Tavistock Clinic Pre-selection Series*	47	(70)	20	(30)
Staunton Clinic Non-selection	34	(65)	18	(35)
Cassel Hospital Limited Interview	24	(55)	20	(45)
Frankfurt Institute Selection	2	(22)	7	(78)
Tavistock Clinic Post-selection Series I*	42	(39)	66	(61)
Tavistock Clinic Post-selection Series II	16	(38)	26	(62)

* Omitting Class X

The table convincingly demonstrates the positive correlation between the Mutual Selection Interview and 'success' in a Balint-type Training Scheme. The correlation seems to hold true over different schemes in different countries.

CHAPTER 7

Factors Affecting Success of Training
by Peter Hildebrand

---

1. THE MUTUAL SELECTION INTERVIEW AS A PREDICTOR

In Chapter 6 we demonstrated the value of the Mutual Selection Interview in increasing the proportion of doctors to whom the Training Scheme gave an experience that proved to be worthwhile for the Scheme and rewarding for the doctor. In this chapter we examine the possibility of correlating the categories used in rating the Mutual Selection Interview with eventual 'success' or 'failure' in the Scheme.[1]

When we began this study, we were still using Michael Balint's empirical formulation that unless a doctor stayed at least a year in one of our seminars, the limited change in personality which was then considered to be essential for the acquisition of psychological skills was unlikely to have taken place. I originally suggested that we call all doctors staying more than a year 'successes' and those who stayed less than a year 'failures'. This suggestion was not accepted by my colleagues because they felt that the time factor, while necessary, was not sufficient to explain the changes that took place

[1] 'Success' and 'failure' are defined in Chapter 4, pp. 49–55, and Chapter 6, pp. 71–73.

90

in the doctors. However, I felt that it might be worth trying, but I found that the categories which had thrown up significant differences between the 'convergent' and 'divergent' groups at selection (see *Table 6*) did not enable us to distinguish between doctors who stayed less than a year and those who stayed longer. It is noteworthy that this extended even to the psychiatrist's prediction about each doctor. While it is true that psychiatrists were not specifically asked to predict success or failure, or even length of attendance, prediction is an integral part of the Mutual Selection Interview. However, when I tried to infer from the notes, I found that the predictive value of the interviews was nil in terms of the length of time that a doctor actually stayed on the course.

In reviewing our work we noted that a major difficulty was the general flatness of the tone of the notes in this convergent group of doctors. I felt that this might well be the effect of the psychiatrist's ambivalence – that he would tend to make allowances for a poor relationship and note it as being more promising than it was in fact, while being rather guarded about a good relationship and seeking possible difficulties in the case of a promising applicant. Moreover, when I rated the records of the interviews, I found that I gave a far more guarded prediction than the psychiatrists. Of course, I had neither the advantage nor the disadvantage of actual personal contact with the applicant. I found that I tended to concentrate most of my attention on factors that would indicate potential failure, as these were far more easily isolated than were those which might predict success. After discussing this difficulty with my colleagues, we agreed that an important variable, which was not at that time being recorded, might be the warmth and empathy which each individual doctor brought to the Mutual Selection Interview and to the particular psychiatrist concerned. We felt, moreover, that an additional factor might be that the psychiatrist's interest

91

and enthusiasm for the course might well have obscured difficulties for the individual doctor that would re-emerge when
he met his seminar and leader for the first time.

Despite this difficulty, we decided to correlate the Mutual
Selection Interview categories with each doctor's eventual
rating on the rating scale. When we used the rating scale,
we got results that correlated positively with the selection
categories, and the proportion of poor predictions dropped
considerably. The results are set out in *Table 12* below.

TABLE 12. CONVERGENT GROUP

COMPARISON OF 'FAILURES' WITH 'SUCCESSES'
IN TERMS OF SELECTION CATEGORIES

	'Failures' (A–D$_1$)		'Successes' (D$_2$–F)	
	No.	*%*	*No.*	*%*
Number of doctors	29		41	
Signs of disturbance:				
present	8	(28)	8	(20)
absent	21		33	
Ordinary confusion:				
present	5	(17)	10	(24)
absent	24		31	
Clear impression of self and practice:				
present	21	(72)	32	(78)
absent	8		9	
Awareness of psychiatric needs:				
in self, present	17	(59)	22	(54)
in practice, present	3	(10)	7	(17)
Lack of awareness:	3	(10)	2	(5)
Communication: good	9	(31)	21	(51)
poor	7	(24)	3	(7)
Evasiveness	5	(17)	4	(10)
Prediction: good	14	(48)	25	(61)
poor	7	(24)	8	(20)
nil	8	(28)	6	(15)

In particular I found that the proportion of wrong predictions dropped, and the ability to communicate freely about oneself and others and make a real contact with the psychiatrist correlated with 'success' as rated on the scale. While we found no significant differences between the 'failures' and the 'successes', it was remarkable that in each case the proportion of 'successes' scoring on the awareness, good communication, lack of disturbance categories was always higher than those of the 'failures'. In no case were the 'failures' given better scores in these categories than the 'successes'. The consistency of these results is impressive and suggests that with better recording the differences between the two groups would be statistically significant. In the present study it is not really surprising that differences of such a magnitude did not arise since the interviews took place before we devised the rating scale and were not recorded with the aim of elucidating these particular qualities. We would infer that the effect of the Mutual Selection Interview has been to increase the proportion of doctors who both the observer and the psychiatrist felt would be aware, flexible, able to communicate about themselves and others, and reasonably secure in themselves.

2. OTHER POSSIBLE FACTORS AFFECTING SUCCESS OF TRAINING

While it was plain that selection was contributing to better results, we agreed that it was necessary to try to exclude the possibility that other factors might have played a part in determining whether a doctor was an early leaver or a stayer, a 'failure' or a 'success'. One possibility that we recognized from the beginning was that, after the hard work and excitement of the pioneering days, we might in the Post-selection phases have been recruiting a special group of highly trained, psychologically skilled doctors whose pro-longed participation depended particularly on such qualities as youth, better training, higher intelligence, etc.

In the present study we have confined ourselves to such information about our medical colleagues as was common knowledge and have not asked them to fill in questionnaires about themselves and their attitudes. This restriction on our inquiries meant that we had no record even of the ages of our doctors when they joined the course. We have used instead the year of qualification as listed in the *Medical Directory*.[1] Unfortunately, approximately 12 per cent. of the doctors were not listed in this publication, so our figures are not complete. The 195 doctors for whom we have this informa-tion had been qualified for between one and fifty-two years when they first came to us. The mean length of time after qualification was fifteen years; but this is rather high be-cause there was a high proportion of elderly doctors accepted in the early Pre-selection phase of the Scheme and this has boosted the average. It seems more important that roughly 60 per cent. of our doctors came in their 5th–15th year after qualification. The mode – the most frequently found figure – was at six years after qualification.

In *Table 13* we set out a comparison between length of time since qualification versus rating on the scale. For ease of computation we have taken length of time since qualifica-tion in decades.

As will be clear from the table, fifty-five out of eighty-one of the practitioners coming to the Scheme in their first ten years after qualification were able to use the seminars pro-ductively. This is slightly more than two-thirds of the sample. In the next decade the proportion falls to exactly 50 per cent. and then gradually decreases with length of time after qualification. Rather more than two-thirds of those practi-

[1] A private directory and not the official Medical Register.

TABLE 13. YEARS SINCE QUALIFICATION CORRELATED WITH RATINGS ON SCALE

Years since Qualification	'Failure' Ratings					'Success' Ratings				
	$A+X+B$	$C_1 \& C_2$	$C_3 \& C_4$	D_1	Sub-Total	D_2	E	F	Sub-Total	Total
1–10	11	4	3	8	26	22	23	10	55	81
11–20	7	8	6	10	31	15	10	6	31	62
21–30	6	2	5	9	22	9	6	2	17	39
31–52	3	2	2	2	9	2	2	–	4	13
Sub-total	27	16	16	29		48	41	18		195
No record	13	2	7	1		–	5	–		28
Total	40	18	23	30		48	46	18		223

tioners for whom we have data come in the first twenty years after qualification, and it is in this group that the majority of 'successes' are to be found. These doctors seem to be able to attach themselves more freely to the seminar and to the new ways of looking at their working with the doctor–patient relationship, which they could discuss with their colleagues. We feel that for men in their 30s and early 40s the Scheme is a most valuable postgraduate training experience.

We also noted, however, that 40 per cent. of the older doctors who came to the Scheme were found to have been rated as having stayed and improved their skills. A very small proportion of these reached the F rating, only two out of twenty-one; but for a doctor in his 50s an increase in his capacity to appreciate the subtleties of the doctor–patient relationship, while it might not reach beyond a D_2 level, could be as considerable an achievement as an F rating for a younger man. Thus we did not feel we were attracting an unduly high proportion of young doctors nor, indeed, that successful participation in the Scheme was solely the province of the doctor in his 30s.

In the next table we show that the institution of the Mutual Selection Interview seems to have screened out those elderly doctors who were set in their ways and found the course unsympathetic. *Table 14* compares the Pre-selection sample with the Post-selection samples in terms of years since qualification.

Inspection of *Table 14* shows that before selection procedures were instituted approximately 40 per cent. of the doctors joining the course had qualified at least twenty-one years before entry. This figure is almost halved, dropping to 22 per cent. after 1956. It seems plain that selection has screened out a proportion of elderly doctors, but that it has not screened out those doctors who could use the course.

We also considered the possibility that the interest shown

96

TABLE 14. DATE OF ENTRY VERSUS YEARS
SINCE QUALIFICATION

	Years since qualification				
	1–10	*11–20*	*21–30*	*31+*	*Total*
Pre-selection 1951–6	25	15	18	7	65
Percentage of Pre-selection Series	(38%)	(23%)	(28%)	(11%)	
Post-selection 1956 and after	56	47	21	6	130
Percentage of Post-selection Series	(43%)	(36%)	(16%)	(5%)	
				Not known	28
					223

in the Tavistock Scheme after the publication of Balint's book had attracted a particularly intelligent and well-trained type of doctor. Certainly when examined we found that two out of three had taken university medical qualifications rather than Conjoint. Moreover, one out of three of our doctors had taken the trouble to obtain either such minor diplomas relevant to general practice as the Diploma in Obstetrics, the Diploma in Child Health, the Diploma in Public Health, etc., and in a few cases held such higher qualifications as Membership of the Royal College of Physicians, the Diploma in Psychological Medicine, or a Doctorate in Philosophy. Although we understand that the College of General Practitioners is proposing to publish a survey of the qualifications of general practitioners, at the time of writing this is not yet available so that we cannot say whether this is significantly higher than either the National or the London average.

About 10 per cent. of our doctors were women. We compared ratings in Post-selection Series I to see whether men or women achieved significantly higher ratings as a group. We could find absolutely no evidence for superiority, whether masculine or feminine, so that it seems that the sex of the doctor makes no difference to his or her ability to acquire psychological skills.

3. THE EXPERIENCE OF THE SEMINAR LEADER

We have also examined the effect of the degree of experience of the seminar leader on the doctor's ultimate rating. As Michael Balint points out in Chapter 3, most training courses in psychological medicine have acted on the unconfirmed principle that any refresher course given by a bona fide specialist is suitable for any general practitioner. In our Scheme, on the other hand, we make the condition that well-trained psychiatrists who are also psycho-analysts should spend a period of at least a year in observing and participating in at least two seminars before they are asked to lead their own seminars. To our surprise we found that even after this long apprenticeship the proportion of doctors leaving in the first year in the initial seminar taken by an inexperienced leader is significantly greater than the proportion leaving in the first year of seminars started by experienced leaders. If we used each psychiatrist as his own control we found that the proportion of doctors staying longer than a year is significantly higher in the psychiatrist's subsequent seminars than in his initial one. It seems that every leader, like everyone else, has to learn a new skill. He needs to come to terms both with the anxiety inherent in leading general practitioner seminars and with the calls made on him by the participants for various types of relationship. Until he has had the opportunity of working these problems through and has had the bitter experience of losing some members of his seminar as a result of his mistakes, he cannot function as effectively as a more experienced leader. We ourselves prefer to talk of a period of in-service training lasting from two to three years before even experienced leaders acquire the necessary skill to lead a general practitioner seminar effectively.

In *Table 15* we have set out the figures comparing the leader's first seminar with his subsequent seminars in Post-selection Series I.

TABLE 15. POST-SELECTION SERIES I

	A	B	C_1	C_2	C_3	C_4	D_1	D_2	E	F	Total
1st seminar	1	3	2	–	2	6	11	7	10	3	45
Subsequent seminars	5	1	1	4	–	3	3	19	18	9	63
							Doctor rated X				1
											109

There are several very striking facts about this table. If we leave out those doctors who attended for only a limited time, rated A, and the one doctor rated X, the number of doctors leaving in the first year of a leaders' first seminar is thirteen (29 per cent.) compared with nine (15 per cent.) in the case of the more experienced leader. As we have already shown in Chapter 6 doctors falling into the C_3 and C_4 classes are those whom we regard as acceptable risks and it is these doctors who make up most of the casualties with the inexperienced leader. This would suggest that these casualties are due more to a failure of training and inexperience on the part of the seminar leader than to a failure of selection.

It seems clear that as doctors are offered vacancies in new seminars in the order in which they apply to the Clinic, and as it is a matter of chance which leader is free to begin a new seminar, the degree of experience of the leader of their initial seminar will be an important factor in determining whether they leave early or stay for more than a year. Confirmation of this can be found in *Table 16*, where we have tested the significance of the correlation between the experience of the psychiatrist leading the doctor's initial seminar and the eventual rating achieved by the same doctor.

TABLE 16. POST-SELECTION SERIES I
COMPARISON OF LEADER'S EXPERIENCE WITH EVENTUAL OUTCOME

	$B-D_1$	D_2-F	Total
Leader's first seminar	24	20	44
Leader's subsequent seminars	12	46	58
Sub-total			102
A + X			7
Total			109

$\chi^2 = 8\cdot691$, which is significant beyond the $\cdot01$ level

The importance of this table is that it brings into question the efficacy of the Mutual Selection Interview. It is possible that the explanation of the increase in the proportion of better results or 'successes' among doctors attending the course after the Selection Interview was introduced is that the skill of the seminar leader had greatly increased rather than the selection had enabled us to screen out doctors with whom we could not work. I felt that this null hypothesis should be given all available support in order that its disproof should be the more convincing. Such evidence as we had lay mostly in the predictions inferred from the records of the Mutual Selection Interviews. Where the psychiatrist at the interview had been enthusiastic about the chances of a doctor who had, nevertheless, left before a year was out, we found that in nine out of fourteen cases these doctors had begun in a leader's first seminar. On the other hand, there were eight cases where the psychiatrist had been very reserved in his prediction and the doctor had remained for

100

more than a year in a seminar and thus achieved a rating of D_1 or better. All eight doctors had begun with a very experienced seminar leader. While obviously these findings might be challenged on the ground that they rested on the psychologist's judgement, there was some evidence here that it was the experience of the seminar leader that had had a vital effect upon the career of the doctor in his contact with our Scheme rather than the efficiency of the Mutual Selection Interview. The question therefore was whether the improvement in our results was not due more to the increased skill of the seminar leaders than to any effect of the Mutual Selection Interview. Some supporting evidence could be put forward that in some cases the predictions derived from the Mutual Selection Interview had been falsified by the experience of the seminar leader.

We tested this hypothesis in the following manner. We set out in *Table 17* the ratings of all doctors who began in a seminar led by Michael Balint.

TABLE 17. ALL GENERAL PRACTITIONERS BEGINNING IN A SEMINAR WITH MICHAEL BALINT

	A	B	C	D_1	D_2	E	F	Total
Pre-selection								
Seminars (1950–2)	5	7	8	5	2	3	5	35
Seminars (1954–6)	3	1	5	6	3	4	1	23
Post-selection								
Seminars (1956–61)	1	–	3	–	7	15	7	33
								91

Balint began the first seminar in 1950 and the period covered by other seminars covers some four years. By the time he started the next seminars in 1954–6 he had established his training method and had begun the publication of a series of papers in the medical literature. Thus the seminars in

1954–6 were started by an experienced leader who had devoted an enormous amount of time and thought to the method he was employing. Despite this, only 35 per cent. of the doctors in these seminars were 'successes'. Among the short stayers were four doctors rated as C_1 ('seriously neurotic') and one doctor rated as A_2 (not enough intelligence available). Six of the doctors, or 25 per cent., starting in this period were rated D_1. The seminars were organized before the Mutual Selection Interview was established, which is the only factor which differentiates them from the seminars started in 1956 and 1961.

The Post-selection seminars present a remarkably different picture. Although the leader and the procedures are the same, the percentage of doctors who stay for a long period and increase their skills rises to twenty-nine out of thirty-three or 90 per cent. of the sample. In the D_1 class (those who stay a long time but cannot use the course) there are no doctors, compared to 25 per cent. in the earlier sample. Since all these doctors participated in the Mutual Selection Interview we can discount any notion that the greater length of stay and increased skill after selection procedures were established was due only to the leader's increased experience.

It might also be objected that the increase in the proportion of 'successes' after the Mutual Selection Interview was introduced was attributable to the increased skill of one leader, Michael Balint. This objection can be quickly dismissed. If we exclude the doctors who began in seminars led by Michael Balint from our Post-selection Series I, we find that 53 per cent. of the doctors attending the course were successful. After Balint's retirement, when the older leaders had become more experienced, the figure rises to 62 per cent. of all doctors joining the course. The difference, however, is not significant.

4. DISCUSSION

In this chapter we have tried to correlate some features of the Mutual Selection Interview with the 'success' or 'failure' of the individual doctor in the Scheme. In the previous chapter we found that although we could use the interview records to distinguish groups of 'convergent' and 'divergent' doctors, we could not use them to distinguish early leavers from long stayers and 'successes' from 'failures'. We are not surprised at this finding because during the period under review we had not devised a method of recording our interviews that would underline those factors which we felt to be highly correlated with long stay in the course and the acquisition of psychological skills.[1]

However, we were gratified to find that such differences as were observed in the Mutual Selection Interview records seemed to be correlated with the doctor being able to use the course and to work in the seminars. In particular they suggested that empathy, and the capacity to communicate about experience with patients and other people shown at the Mutual Selection Interview, seemed to be the major factors. While we could not draw firm conclusions from this evidence, we tried to test our data in other ways. As we had not wished to subject our colleagues to the sort of interview appropriate for an applicant for a job, we had no information about them beyond that volunteered in the interview or publicly known; but it did seem that such factors as qualifications, sex, etc., made no difference as to whether a

[1] The Interview Recording Form devised by Gosling and Hildebrand on the basis of the present study will be found in Appendix I. This is based on some procedures of the Focal Therapy Workshop (Malan, 1964). This form is now routinely used to record all interviews for courses for general practitioners both at the Tavistock Clinic and at University College Hospital, London. It is hoped to present a study of the results using this form when we have accumulated sufficient numbers.

doctor was an early leaver or a long stayer, a 'success' or a 'failure'. We did, however, find there was a high correlation between the experience of the leader of the doctor's first seminar and the length of stay and eventual rating of the doctor. This factor tended to reduce the value of the selection interview as a predictor of long stay. However, comparison made on the work of one psychiatrist experienced in leading groups, both pre- and post-selection, demonstrated that the leader's skill and experience alone did not account for the success rate.

We have shown that a selection procedure can increase the proportion of successes to a highly acceptable figure. We feel that we now have the basis for a record form which will enable us to correlate with a fair degree of accuracy the characteristics shown by the doctor in the Mutual Selection Interview and his later performance in the seminars. But we also recognize that a good interview and good material may well be vitiated by our need to give leaders in-service training in our Scheme. At present we see no way round this difficulty, although we now invite all doctors leaving the course to a terminal interview and, where possible, offer those who seem to be training casualties alternative vacancies in more promising seminars.

It seems we shall probably continue to lose something like one in four doctors of those who start in a seminar after having been exposed to the Mutual Selection Interview. This figure is related to a combination of two factors: we accept some doctors knowing that they may well turn out to be casualties, and some doctors become 'failures' due to the inexperience of our seminar leaders. The latter are the casualties caused by our use of in-service training methods. We recognize that this proportion of losses might be reduced by the introduction of questionnaires, ability tests, etc., but however desirable this might be from a strictly psychological point of view, our medical colleagues feel that this would destroy the basis of mutual trust and cooperation with which they work with general practitioners. We hope that it will now be possible to devise some new ways of reducing our failure rate but, in the meantime, we feel that, despite these failures, we have made a reasonably satisfying beginning.

CHAPTER 8

Conclusions *by* Michael Balint

WE started this study with two parallel aims in mind. On the one hand, we wished to find out in what way the introduction of the Mutual Selection Interview had influenced our results. On the other hand, we required to know what the real results of our Training Scheme were; what proportion of the participating general practitioners could benefit from it; and whether our methods, judged by our results, had improved in recent years. As always happens in a research, we became involved in many more problems than we had intended. Here I shall attempt a discussion of only the most important results.

1. THE RESULTS OF THE MUTUAL SELECTION INTERVIEW

Let us start with the influence of the Mutual Selection procedure. In *Table 18*, which is a condensed form of *Table 4* in Chapter 6, I have contrasted the distribution of doctors according to our rating scale in the Pre-selection Series with that of the Post-selection Series. At first sight the changes seem to be relevant and all in the right direction.

Any selection has two aspects, negative and positive.

It is difficult to say with certainty whether we succeeded in selecting, positively, the right people as we could not observe

106

TABLE 18. COMPARISON OF RATINGS OF PRE-
AND POST-SELECTION SERIES

Series	A & X %	B %	C_1 & C_2 %	C_3 & C_4 %	D_1 %	D_2 %	E %	F %	Total %
Pre-selection	18	18	14	7	15	8	12	8	100
Post-selection I and II	6	3	5	13	12	28	25	8	100

the development of the doctors who withdrew after the Mutual Selection Interview and, therefore, we have no controls. Still we have a few suggestive facts. It is certain that after the introduction of the Mutual Selection Interview a higher proportion of doctors were able to stay longer, which means that more had better opportunities to acquire the necessary skills. We can see from *Table 18* that the percentage of long stayers, that is Classes D_1 to F, rose from 43 per cent. in the Pre-selection period to 73 per cent. in the Post-selection period.

The other fact also suggesting that we have selected the right people is that among the long stayers, especially with experienced seminar leaders, the proportion of doctors belonging to Class D_1 steadily declined and parallel with it the proportion of Classes D_2 to F steadily increased. The global ratio D_2–F : D_1 was about 2 : 1 in the Pre-selection period and it rose to almost 5 : 1 in the Post-selection period.

The opposite question is whether the Mutual Selection Interview had selected out, negatively, the doubtful or unpromising entrants. Here again we have a few facts to indicate that it might have been so. In the two Post-selection Series there are no doctors rated A_2, that is those who gave the impression of not having enough available intelligence; while the numbers in classes A and X (from 18 per cent. to 6 per cent.), B (from 18 per cent. to 3 per cent.), C_1 and C_2 (from 14 per

107

cent. to 5 per cent.), and D_1 (from 15 per cent. to 12 per cent.) have been considerably reduced.

True, the percentage in Classes C_3 and C_4 has also increased, but this was according to our plan. We consider these doctors as acceptable risks and we deliberately accepted some doubtful applicants in the hope that some of them might be able to benefit from their attendance in spite of our equivocal prediction.

However, to appreciate the real significance of our figures we must take into account the influence of the Mutual Selection Interview. Its effect is to enable doctors who otherwise would have been early leavers to withdraw either at the time of the interview, or some time after, but before the seminar starts. The figures presented in Chapter 6 suggest that this withdrawal cuts out about 40 per cent. of all the applicants. In fact a recent series of interviews conducted in 1964, that is, after we had arrived at the main results of our study, yielded almost exactly the same percentage. I interviewed thirty-one doctors of whom twenty-three agreed to join the course, while eight withdrew (three of them were 'superior' doctors, two belonged to Class C_4, i.e. were over-anxious, two were not actually in general practice, and one was participating in another training scheme). Before starting the seminars one withdrew because he decided to train as a psychiatrist, and four more withdrew in circumstances strongly suggestive of Class C_5, the over-well defended. Thus of the thirty-one original applicants, thirteen were cut out by the Mutual Selection Interview, a loss of 42 per cent., which agrees well with the figures found in our study.

The next question is how to apportion the cut of 40 per cent. among the various classes of our rating scale. Our aim with the interview was, as stated on several occasions, to enable doctors who otherwise would be 'early leavers' to withdraw before committing themselves. In the first instance, this means doctors rated as A and X, B, and C_1 and C_2. So let us suppose as a first approximation that all the 40 per cent. should be deducted from these classes in about equal proportions; this would mean 14 per cent. each of the first two classes and 12 per cent. of the third. The resulting distribution is shown in *Table 19*, which in fact is *Table 18* turned vertical.

TABLE 19. COMPARISON OF PRE- AND POST-
SELECTION SERIES AFTER ALLOWING FOR
THE EFFECT OF THE MUTUAL SELECTION
INTERVIEW

Rating	Pre-selection	Cut by Mutual Selection Interview		Calculated percentages	Actual percentages in Post-selection Series I & II	Difference
1	% *2*	% *3*	*4*	% *5*	% *6*	% *7*
A & X	18	−14 =	4	→7	6	−1
B	18	−14 =	4	→7	3	−4
C_1 & C_2	14	−12 =	2	→3	5	+2
C_3 & C_4	7		7	→12	13	+1
D_1	15		15	→25	12	−13
D_2	8		8	→13	28	+15
E	12		12	→20	25	+5
F	8		8	→13	8	−5
Total	100	−40 =	60	→100	100	
Absolute figure	72				151	

Its fourth column shows the distribution of percentages calculated on this basis; in order to make it comparable with the percentages actually found in Post-selection Series I and II, these figures, which add up to sixty, had to be recalculated so that their respective proportions should remain the same but their sum total should make 100. These latter figures are shown in column 5. In column 6 we have printed for comparison the actual percentages of Post-selection Series I and II and, lastly, in column 7 the differences between the calculated figures and the figures actually found.

This table shows clearly the results of our Mutual Selection Interview. The numbers in the classes containing the doctors who are highly unlikely to benefit from our sort of training have considerably diminished; Class B, that is, those doctors whom we could not diagnose at all, has diminished still more than predicted. In contrast the numbers in Classes C_3 and C_4, our acceptable risks, have remained as predicted, or even slightly higher. Thus there can be no question that the Mutual Selection Interview has served its purpose. Moreover, if we disregard the 13 per cent. of the population attributable to Classes C_3 and C_4, our acceptable risks, there remains only 14 per cent. – that is, 6 per cent. in Classes A and X, 3 per cent. in Class B, and 5 per cent. in Classes C_1 and C_2 – which can be considered as failures of selection. This means one in seven, or one in eight, which is a commendable result.

2. THE RESULTS OF THE TRAINING

The next task will be to consider in detail the results of our Training Scheme. Taking first *Table 18*, we may proudly point out that while the percentage in Class D_1 has been slightly reduced from 15 per cent. to 12 per cent., the figures in D_2 and E have increased impressively and, lastly, the figures in Class F have remained unchanged. However, before we draw any far-reaching conclusions from these figures, we ought to remind ourselves that any change in them may be attributed to two causes: (*a*) the influence of the Mutual Selection Interview, and (*b*) the improvement of our training methods.

So let us now turn to *Table 19* in which we tried to eliminate the changes brought about by the Mutual Selection Interview, which, as explained in the previous section, acts by cutting out about 40 per cent. of the applicants. If we study the bottom half of that table, that is, the figures pertaining to Classes D_1 to F, two important features emerge. One is that the percentage in Class F, instead of remaining constant has, in fact, decreased during the years. On the other hand, the percentage in Class E has increased by the same amount. One explanation of this finding may be that, to reach the level of F, doctors may need some considerable time. This was not available for doctors in Post-selection Series II which was rated after only four terms of attendance. We shall return to discuss this important hypothesis in the next section.

Another hypothesis is that perhaps the proportion of doctors who are able to reach the level of skill required for E or F is, in any population, limited. There is nothing novel in this idea; for instance, everyone would agree that the proportion of doctors who might be trained to be first-rate surgeons, would prove to be limited. This hypothesis will be discussed in Section 5.

The other important feature is the definite decrease in the number of doctors rated D_1, i.e. those in whose cases our training methods proved ineffective in spite of the doctors' long attendance, and an almost equal increase in the number of doctors rated D_2, i.e. those who showed minimal but significant changes under the influence of the training. This is a relevant finding because it shows that our training methods have improved, in fact, as a comparison of the figures of

111

Post-selection Series I and Series II shows, are still improving.

We must not forget, however, that *Table 19* is based on global figures, that is, on the results of all the psychiatrists taking part in our Training Scheme, no matter whether they are beginners or experienced. As has been already shown in Chapter 7, there are significant differences between their achievements. This will be discussed further in Section 4.

3. THE TIME FACTOR

The next question is that of the influence of time. *Table 20* shows the distribution of our whole population, that is of 223 doctors, according to their length of stay as the first variable (see Chapter 4, p. 43) and their rating as the second variable (see Chapter 4, pp. 44–57).

TABLE 20. RATING VERSUS LENGTH OF STAY

Length of Stay	Rating											Total
	X	A	B	C_1	C_2	C_3	C_4	D_1	D_2	E	F	
Class I	5	15	16	9	8	8	13	–	2	4	–	80
Class II	–	1	2	–	1	–	2	8	7	8	1	30
Class III								6	1	6	1	14
Class IV								1	8	5	8	22
Still attending								13	28	21	5	67
Transfer	1							2	2	2	3	10
	6	16	18	9	9	8	15	30	48	46	18	223

As expected, most of the doctors belonging to Classes X to C_4 stayed less than one year and only very few as long as two. Since, as discussed in Chapter 4, this half of the table cannot but repeat what we have put into it, it cannot teach us anything new. The other half of the table, that is, Classes D_1 to

F, shows a rather irregular distribution, one reason for which is the comparatively high number of doctors in 'Still Attending' and 'Transfer'. In order to eliminate their disturbing influence, we ascertained the length of stay of each doctor in these two classes and classified him accordingly.

TABLE 21. DOCTORS RATED D_1-F VERSUS
RECLASSIFIED LENGTH OF STAY

Reclassified length of Stay	Rating								Total
	D_1		D_2		E		F		
	No.	%	No.	%	No.	%	No.	%	
Class I	–	–	2	–	4	–	–	–	6
Class II	11		15		14		1		41
		27		37		34		2	
Class III	8		7		12		1		28
		29		25		43		4	
Class IV	11		24		16		16		67
		16		36		24		24	
Total	30		48		46		18		142
Total of classes X–C_4									81
Grand total									223

Table 21 shows the resulting figures restricted to the relevant classes, i.e. D_1 to F. In each cell the absolute figure is printed in the top left-hand corner, while the percentage is in the bottom right-hand corner.

Because they are small, I propose to disregard the figures of Class I, that is, those doctors who left during their first year of attendance. One could even lump them together with Class II because all the six doctors, two in D_2 and four in E, left at the end of their first year, but before they started their

113

second year. In some ways this procedure could be justified, but it would detract from the clarity of the picture.

The trend among the remaining figures is quite clear. The percentage of D_1 doctors remains constant in Classes II and III at 27 per cent. to 29 per cent. and drops suddenly in Class IV, that is, for those doctors who stayed longer than three years, to 16 per cent. On the other hand the proportion of doctors rated D_2 seems to remain fairly constant at 36 per cent. to 37 per cent. True, there is a drop in Class III to 25 per cent., but I think this is caused partly by the smallness of the absolute figure – only seven – in this cell, and partly possibly to uncertainties in the classification, as mentioned in Chapter 5. It is certainly not without significance that in the same Class III the number of E doctors shows a sudden jump from about 30 per cent. to 43 per cent. To smooth down these two irregularities in the curves we need only to assume that two to three doctors who ought to belong to Class D_2 were somewhat sympathetically rated as E.

But even if we refrain from smoothing our curves, it is clear from *Table 21* that the percentage of doctors rated as E falls sharply in Class IV from *circa* 34 per cent. to 24 per cent. and, at the same time, the proportion of the doctors rated as F rises equally sharply from 4 per cent. to 24 per cent. This important finding is statistically significant. It gives support to our impression, which formed one of the bases for our rating scale, that doctors belonging to Class D_1 do not seem to have the potential for considerable development. Something similar holds true for some of the doctors rated D_2. On the other hand a proportion of those initially rated D_2 move, at the end of the first or the second year, up to E or even to F. And lastly, the same seems to be true for doctors rated as E.

Conversely this means that, in order to achieve a rating of F, most doctors need considerable time. The critical period seems to be their third year. Roughly one-quarter of the doctors who could commit themselves enough to stay longer than three years develop so far that they are rated F. In the discussion of *Table 18* this influence of time on the rating was mentioned as a possible factor.

4. THE EXPERIENCE OF THE STAFF

As mentioned in the beginning of Section 2, the Mutual Selection Interview, which was introduced in 1956, has considerably improved the results of our Training Scheme. Its main effect was to allow about 40 per cent. of the applicants to withdraw either at the interview itself or in the period between the interview and the start of the seminar. In Chapters 6 and 7, Peter Hildebrand has discussed in detail the reasons why we think that these 'divergent' doctors are those who in any case would be unlikely to stay sufficiently long in the training. Thus the first effect of the Mutual Selection Interview has been to free the training from these doctors.

However, as anyone who has had some experience with groups knows, any member who leaves represents a trauma to the rest of the group. The Mutual Selection Interview, by cutting down the number of early leavers, detraumatized, so to speak, the later seminars to a considerable degree and thus secured for them a smoother development. Our present study does not allow us to prove this assumption by figures; nevertheless it rests on rather convincing impressions.

A corollary to this change is a changed direction of attention in the leader, especially in the beginner. Losing a member of his group is always felt as a failure by the leader. Each loss initiates in him an anxious scrutiny of his methods which, as a rule, has an inhibiting effect on him. If his 'failures' are less numerous, he can develop more freely.

That this sort of development in fact takes place is

convincingly shown in Chapter 7. To illustrate it, I repro-
duce here *Table 16* from that chapter as *Table 22.*

TABLE 22.* POST-SELECTION SERIES I

COMPARISON OF LEADER'S EXPERIENCE WITH
EVENTUAL OUTCOME

	$B-D_1$	D_2-F	*Total*
Leader's first seminar	24	20	44
Leader's subsequent seminars	12	46	58
Sub-total	36	66	102
A and X			7
Total			109

* Repetition of *Table 16*

We used for this demonstration Post-selection Series I.
First, a number of psychiatrists began their career as leader
during this period and, second, we had a sufficiently long
time to observe the results and are thus fairly confident that
our observations are reliable. *Table 22* shows that the beginners had about as many 'failures' as 'successes', while the
ratio for the experienced leaders was about one to four. However, these figures are still global; they include all the beginners and all the experienced leaders and, further, they do not
differentiate between the early and the later stages of the
development of any particular leader.

To show what this means, we constructed *Table 23*, which
is a condensed version of *Table 21* in Chapter 7 about the
ultimate ratings of all the doctors who started their career in
the Training Scheme with me.

This table shows the influences of increasing experience on
the one hand and of the Mutual Selection Interview on the
other, as has already been pointed out in Chapter 7. In the
very first period, before gaining much experience in how to
116

TABLE 23. EVENTUAL OUTCOME OF DOCTORS
STARTING WITH MICHAEL BALINT

	$B-D_1$	D_2-F	Total
Pre-selection			
Seminars (1950–2)	20	10	30
Seminars (1954–6)	12	8	20
Post-selection			
Seminars (1956–61)	3	29	32
Sub-total			82
A			9
Total			91

lead a training group, I had more 'failures' than 'successes'.
In the second period, after a proper training method had been
worked out in the research with my 'Old Guard', there were
about as many 'successes' as 'failures', with a slight prepon-
derance of the latter. Lastly, in the later periods, when the
influences of increased experience and the Mutual Selection
Interview reinforced each other, the proportion of 'failures'
was reduced to about 10 per cent. of the total.

This has been for all of us a highly disquieting finding. We
always believed that, no matter how well a psychiatrist had
been trained, he had to learn the art of leading a training
seminar. Acting on this belief, we laid down, on a purely
empirical basis, that he should attend at least two seminars,
each for a minimum period of six months. The statistical
evidence raises this belief to the status of a proven fact, but
also shows that our stringent conditions have not been
stringent enough. Even after psycho-analytic training, and
some considerable experience in psychiatry as well as of being
an observer in training seminars, the new leaders achieve
significantly poorer results than do the experienced ones.
A difficult dilemma arises here. Can we accept responsibility
for exposing the general practitioners to considerably reduced
chances of success with an inexperienced leader? If not, how

1

can we meet the ever increasing demand for new leaders of new groups? We must admit that as yet we have not found a satisfactory answer to this problem.

5. OUR APPLICANTS AS A POPULATION

All our attempts at finding out whether doctors who attended our Training Scheme are a representative sample of the population of general practitioners have failed, mainly because, for the time being, there are no reliable statistical data available on this subject. The only thing we know is that the proportion of men to women is about the same in our doctors as among general practitioners. Otherwise, as discussed in Chapters 6 and 7, we know that two out of three of our doctors have a university degree and only one in three a Conjoint Diploma, and further, that about one in three has at least one minor postgraduate diploma relevant to general practice. This means that our sample perhaps belongs to the better-than-average stratum of general practitioners; this however is only a guess.

Another finding that may be important is that about 60 per cent. of our doctors join us between five and fifteen years after their qualification and, on the whole, this group seems to fare better in our rating scale than the remaining 40 per cent. This latter finding might be coupled with an impression that in recent years the number of doctors belonging to the older age group has diminished in comparison with the younger ones. If the impression of this trend proves to be correct, it will have important effects on the overall results of our training.

Though we cannot decide how far the general practitioners who apply for our training are a representative sample of the whole general practitioner population, we have been able to analyse our sample and isolate certain characteristics. In order to assess the importance of these characteristics in their proper proportions, we have to take into account that about 40 per cent. of all the applicants were cut out by the Mutual Selection Interview in our Post-selection Series I and II. To undo this effect we constructed *Table 24*, which in a way is a reversal of *Table 19*. There we had to calculate how the percentages would increase proportionately because of the 40 per cent. cut out by the Mutual Selection Interview; here we have to calculate how the percentages actually found in the Post-selection period would decrease proportionately if we wished to reintroduce the 40 per cent. that had been cut out

TABLE 24. CONSTITUTION OF DIFFERENT MEDICAL POPULATIONS ACCORDING TO THEIR EVENTUAL OUTCOME

	Post-selection Series I and II		*Pre-selection Series*	*Staunton (no selection)*	*Cassel (some selection)*
	Found %	*Calculated* %	*Found* %	*Found* %	*Found* %
A & X	6 →	4	18	8	5
B	3 →	2	18	21	13
C_1 & C_2	5 →	3	15	11	10
C_3 & C_4	12 →	7	6	10	20
D_1	12 →	7	15	15	7
D_2	28 →	17	8	21	15
E	26 →	15	12	10	25
F	8 →	5	8	4	5
	100 →	60	100	100	100
Divergent		25			?
Second thoughts		15			?
		100			

by the Mutual Selection Interview. In the subsequent columns the figures found in the Pre-selection Series by the Staunton Clinic, and by the Cassel Hospital, were added for comparison.

If we add up in the Post-selection Series I and II the 'divergents', that is, the doctors who at the interview decided against joining the Scheme, those who had 'second thoughts', and the early leavers, that is, Classes A–C$_4$, we get 56 per cent. that is, a larger half of the applicants. Remarkably, almost exactly the same figures occur in the Pre-selection Series, 57 per cent. in the Staunton Clinic sample, 50 per cent., while in the Cassel Hospital sample, where there was a very mild form of selection, the figure was 48 per cent. That means that about every other doctor who shows enough interest to apply for the course and to come to the interview finds that his expectations and ours are so far from each other that the only materially acceptable solution that can be found is to part.

Of the remaining half, 7 per cent. of our applicants had to be rated as D$_1$, which means that although they were able to tolerate the seminars we did not consider the results achieved to be satisfactory. The figures for the other series were 15 per cent. each for our Pre-selection Series and for the Staunton Clinic sample, and 7 per cent. for the Cassel Hospital. That leaves 37 per cent., that is, almost two in five of all our applicants, who not only found the work in the seminars congenial but were also able to benefit from it. The corresponding figures are: 28 per cent. for our Pre-selection Series, 35 per cent. for the Staunton Clinic, and 45 per cent. for the Cassel Hospital, which is again somewhat out of line because of its selection procedure. And, lastly, exactly 20 per cent., that is, one in five of all the applicants, attained a rating of E or F, which means that they were able to acquire considerable diagnostic and therapeutic skills, different in nature from, though com-
120

parable with, those expected from a psychiatrist. (This is not the place to discuss this important question. Suffice it to say that the differences are caused chiefly by the setting in which the therapeutic work is carried out.) The figures for E and F were: 20 per cent. for the Pre-selection Series, 14 per cent. for the Staunton Clinic, and 30 per cent. for the Cassel Hospital.

It is well known that most, though not all, general practitioners are selected negatively: that is, those who turn towards general practice do so because for some reason or other they do not feel that they can make the grade as specialists. For the last few decades it has been a hotly debated topic in medical circles whether this trend will increase in momentum and if general practice will disappear almost entirely, or, on the contrary, whether we should be prepared for a vigorous revival of general practice. But whatever the future may bring, the fact remains that the most promising young doctors, if at all possible, try to find a place for themselves in one of the specialities. This means that among general practitioners the proportion of highly talented people will be smaller than among the specialists. Taking this bitter but incontrovertible fact into account, the results of our training, as shown by our figures, seem to be acceptable.

Turning the tables, we may now use our figures as indicators of the possible constitution of the general practitioner population. Evidently there will be some inevitable uncertainty in our conclusions for the reasons enumerated in the beginning of this section. It is impossible to assess how far our 223 doctors constitute a representative sample of the whole population; but even if they were, the sample is much too small, amounting to about 1 per cent. of all the general practitioners in the United Kingdom. We must mention yet another feature that restricts the validity of our conclusions: that is that a good 90 per cent. of our doctors' practices are situated in London or in the Home Counties. And, last, our

121

sample consists entirely of volunteers, the results of a strict self-selection.

All these considerations warn us to be cautious with our inferences. However, we have another finding that suggests that our figures are not due to some chance coincidence, but reveal inherent features of the present-day general practitioner population. What we have found is that our figures are paralleled by those in other centres of medical training where our rating scale was adopted. This important finding has been discussed already in Chapter 6 and is demonstrated again in *Table 24*. While in Chapter 6 Peter Hildebrand reviewed all the material available, in *Table 24* only the samples with large enough absolute figures were included; apart from our two Series, *Table 24* shows the sample of the Cassel Hospital, which is situated in Richmond, a fairly distant suburb of London, which until 1964 was outside the London County Council area, and the sample of the Staunton Clinic, University of Pittsburgh, Pa., U.S.A.

If we disregard the influence of a mild selection procedure which distorts somewhat the Cassel figures, the four Series are almost identical. We may add that we have indications that the situation in Germany is similar, and some impressions that it is the same in Holland, France, and Switzerland – the countries with which we have had sufficiently close contact. Of course these impressions have to be supported by statistical evidence. But even if we restrict ourselves to the evidence already available, we learn that the constitution of the medical population shows marked similarities in various parts of the Western world, and until now no medical community has been found different from this pattern.

These findings have most important consequences for our Training Scheme. To repeat what was stated above: they warn us that about 50 per cent. of the present medical population will find our ideas and methods uncongenial and will not be able to work with us. Another 5 per cent. to 10 per cent. of the population will be able to stay with the Scheme but are apparently unable to benefit much from it; these are our Class D_1. This means that for about 55 per cent. to 60 per cent. of all doctors our offer of training in its present form will prove unacceptable. Most of them do not even feel the need for deepening their psychological understanding of their patients, while those among this group who try will find our aims and methods unhelpful or overexacting. In consequence they either leave us or, if they stay, will not change.

In contrast, for the smaller half, about two-fifths of all the doctors, the seminars are not only tolerable but welcome; they can make proper use of their new experiences. Finally, we can expect that about one half of this last group, almost exactly 20 per cent. of all the doctors, will be able to use the seminars to acquire a commendable amount of diagnostic and therapeutic skill.

It would be interesting to examine the causes and the consequences of this state of affairs. Among the causes, perhaps the most important is the content of present-day medical training, which is entirely in the hands of specialists and is based on the scientific analysis of part functions such as anatomy, physiology, biochemistry, etc., to the detriment of the study of the whole person. The consequences include: the neglect of psychotherapy in all medical teaching by comparison with physical and chemical methods; the enormous sums spent on 'psychiatric' drugs; the 'scientific' orientation of every young doctor who wants to get on in his profession, and so on. This is not the place to discuss these crucial issues, which go well beyond the scope of our study.

6. OUTLOOK

In this section I shall indulge in speculations about what the various findings, considerations, and ideas discussed in the previous sections mean for the future development of our Training Scheme.

The first question on which to speculate is what help we may expect to come to us from outside our Scheme. Perhaps the most important single factor under this heading is the gradual change in the general atmosphere of medical practice. More and more doctors realize not only the immense successes but also the painful limitations of the present-day 'scientific' or 'biological' way of thinking and are converted to thinking in terms of a 'whole-person' medicine. It is to be expected that this trend will influence medical training increasingly in the coming years.

It has been mentioned on several occasions that in recent years the proportion of younger doctors has steadily increased among our applicants; we have got the impression that, parallel with this, fewer and fewer doctors with a pioneering or reformist spirit applied and that we get more and more doctors of the well-trained, ordinary type. Lastly we hope that knowledge about the special nature of our Training Scheme will spread among the medical population, partly by the written and partly by the spoken word, and that this will reduce the proportion of 'divergent' doctors among our applicants.

The second, and much more complicated, question is: what should we try to achieve by research and concentrated effort? Let us start our speculations with the research aspect. One of the first tasks will be to refine our present rating scale. This research will have to be concentrated – as predicted in Chapter 4 – on the borderland between the Classes C and D. On the whole I think that Classes C_1, 'seriously neurotic', and

124

C_2, 'superior', are defined sufficiently exactly and will need but little attention. Class B, 'undiagnosable', has practically disappeared in any case and thus will not need attention either. On the other hand, Class D_1 presents a serious problem. In our scale it is described only clinically as consisting of doctors who can tolerate the seminar but cannot change under its influence. In many respects Class D_1 fulfilled the same function for the stayers as Class B did for the early leavers; it offered an acceptable label for our lack of knowledge. In consequence its future ought to be the same, and its size should be reduced to insignificance. What is needed is a proper study enabling us to diagnose the doctors belonging to Class D_1 properly and to understand their rigidity in dynamic terms. In some cases this better understanding will lead to a change in our methods, while in other cases it will lead to a decision to help these doctors withdraw earlier from an apparently unprofitable venture. Here I wish to recall our findings in Section 3 according to which the proportion of D_1 doctors is considerably diminished after the third year.

This intensive study of the doctors belonging to Class D_1 – and possibly to D_2 also – will influence our somewhat vague ideas about Classes C_3, C_4 and the recently proposed C_5 as defined in Chapter 4, Section 2. The main problem in these three classes will be to work out criteria for differential diagnosis separating those who will almost certainly drop out in the early stages, that is, the real C doctors, from those who with a somewhat modified training method might be able to stay and qualify for a D_2 or E.

The recently isolated Class C_5 will need special attention. First, its characteristic should be more precisely defined so that we should know whether it is justified to establish it as a special group, or whether it would be more realistic to consider it only as a sub-group of Class C_4. In this respect a very important group for study will be the doctors who accept our offer of a place in a seminar but then withdraw before the seminar starts, whom we now call 'second-thought' doctors. What has to be found out is how many of them belong to the new Class C_5.

It is hoped that if all this can be done, that is, the characteristics of the various classes in our rating scale can be more exactly defined, the degree of agreement between the various raters will increase (see Chapter 5).

The second focus of research should be the Mutual Selection Interview. As has just been discussed, the working out of differential diagnostic criteria and a more exact definition of the characteristics of Classes C and D in our rating scale will enable the interviewer to see more clearly and more exactly. I do not think that this will lead to a disappearance of the rare open disagreements in the Mutual Selection Interview – as it will be remembered all these occurred with doctors belonging to Class C_1 – but it may reduce the number of the doctors with 'second thoughts', those accepted under C_3 and especially C_4, and, lastly, those whose ultimate rating was not higher that D_1. On the other hand, a refinement of the Mutual Selection Interview technique might encourage some doctors who withdrew unnecessarily to stay with us. As mentioned in Section 1, we have no opportunity of learning anything about their possible number. And lastly, as discussed in Chapters 6 and 7, an important task will be to develop the Mutual Selection Interview as an instrument of prediction. This research, under the influence of the present study, has already been started both at the Tavistock Clinic and at University College Hospital; the results to date are most encouraging.

A third research project should choose as its object the 'reshuffle' mentioned in Chapters 1 and 2. We described there that after about two years of working together – and losing some of their members – the seminars are disbanded and then regrouped. This occasion has been used: (*a*) to separate, on the whole, the fast from the slow developers or, in terms of the rating scale, to group together the D_1s and D_2s on the one hand, and the Es and Fs on the other; (*b*) to expose the doctors to another leader. We know that in some cases this 're-shuffle' has acted as a powerful stimulus, accelerating the doctor's development; in others it has had an inhibiting effect; in still others no immediate effect has been observed; and lastly, in some cases it has led to the doctor's leaving the Scheme. These highly important effects will need a detailed study.

Another – and very important – piece of research will be to devise a better way of integrating the in-service training of new leaders and the Training Scheme. This, as mentioned in Section 4, is a most difficult problem, and at present we do not even know how to tackle it.

The last, the largest, and by far the most important research problem will be to define the aims and methods of our training in terms of our rating scale.

On the whole it seems that the two most important classes that have emerged after the introduction of the Mutual Selection Interview are D_2 and E, which together make up more than half, exactly 54 per cent., of all entrants into our Scheme. If this trend proves to be real and constant, not influenced, that is, either by the gradual increase of younger doctors among the applicants, or by the increasing experience of the training staff, it will necessitate a rethinking of our aims and methods.

I, for one, thought at first that quite a sizable proportion of general practitioners could – provided they can get training from an experienced group leader – attain a level corresponding to F. Our figures suggest that this was perhaps a much too ambitious view, since 54 per cent. of our doctors in the Post-selection period belong to Classes D_2 and E, while only 8 per cent. are rated as F.

A doctor who is a candidate for F could be described as a 'born' or 'gifted' practitioner, a kind of artist. It is highly probable that he will derive from his professional work enough 'deep' satisfaction to compensate him for the strains caused by the training. In this way he will be able to give up without too much pain some of his accustomed ways of behaving towards his patients and to achieve the often mentioned 'considerable though limited change of his personality'. This idea may explain the ease and willingness in them to accept on approval, so to speak, the new ways and to experiment with them. It is also consistent with the pattern of development typical of them, namely, one of continuous progress right from the start with occasional sudden bursts, as mentioned in Chapter 4.

If I may extend this simile, in contrast to them, doctors belonging to Classes D_2 and E give the impression of confident and sensible craftsmen. What they seem to need is, first, more conviction that what they learn at considerable cost to themselves will be valuable, and then, ample opportunity to acquire these new skills. This is a somewhat different process, not so much a becoming aware of what has already been there in the doctor, but accepting something new that he has not yet possessed and assimilating it to the extent that he can use it with ease, free from being impeded by his new acquisition. The two principal forms in which this lack of freedom presents itself are: (*a*) a feeling that he must do what is expected from him, and (*b*) a crippling fear that, however hard he tries, he will not be able to make the grade.

As I have just admitted, in the preceding years I was more concerned with making the doctors aware of their own resources – such as sensitivity, sympathy, understanding, and so on – than offering them something external to them, and at the same time helping them to cope with the conflicts, fears, and problems that this offer might provoke. If my train of thought is correct, in the coming period we must concentrate our efforts so that we may be able to give better chances to the most important sector of our entrants, the D_2 and E doctors. This will mean a certain shift of emphasis in our training methods, certainly in mine.

For the last flight of my speculation I will try to predict in which direction the results of our Training Scheme may change in the next decade or so. With the improvement of the techniques of our Mutual Selection Interview and the expected change in the general atmosphere, the percentage of the 'divergent' doctors will drop to 10 per cent. to 20 per cent., and those having 'second thoughts' before starting the seminars to about 5 per cent. to 10 per cent. Class B, the doctors whom we cannot diagnose, will practically disappear, and the same will hold true for Classes C_1 and C_2, the doctors unsuitable for our training; all these together will amount to less than 5 per cent. Classes C_3 and C_4 and possibly C_5 – these three classes constitute our acceptable risks – will account for about 10 per cent. of the doctors. And, last, Class D_1 will be considerably reduced, say to about 5 per cent. That would mean that the sum total of all our 'failures' will drop to 30 per cent. to 35 per cent., of which about 20 per cent. will be cut out by the Mutual Selection Interview, while another 10 per cent. to 15 per cent will drop out during their first year of attendance. As mentioned, Class D_1 – our Pass Degree – will be reduced to about 5 per cent. In contrast I expect Class D_2 – our Third Class Honours – to remain at about its present level, or even to increase slightly to about 30 per cent. to 35 per cent., while Classes E and F – our Second and First Class Honours – will account roughly for the remaining 30 per cent., again a considerable increase on our present 20 per cent. How much of this 30 per cent. will qualify for F is difficult to state because it will largely depend on the status of general practice in the future.

129

Mutual Selection Interview

NAME OF APPLICANT: AGE:

NAME OF INTERVIEWER: DATE OF INTERVIEW:

A. *Introduction to Course* (contacts, reading, etc.)

B. (1) *Appearance* of applicant:
   Manner of presenting his application:

   (2) *G.P. problems* and his attitude towards them and to the Course:

   (3) What seems to bring applicant *now*:

C. *Factual material* relevant to application (professional history and status, etc.):

D. (1) Applicant's *conception of himself* as a G.P.:

   (2) Applicant's *conception of other important people*: (partners, competitors, consultants, spouse, etc.)

E. *Developing interviewer/applicant relationship*

   (1) How applicant treated interviewer and any changes in this (in particular, what did applicant do with picture of courses presented by interviewer):

   (2) How interviewer treated applicant and any changes in this:

F. *Important moments in interview*:
   (Points where coherence was disturbed. Personal remarks

made by interviewer and their effect. Perplexing and camouflaging remarks. Specific declarations of anxiety, e.g. 'Are you going to psycho-analyse us?')

G. *Result*

(1) Snap dynamic formulation:
(2) Balint signs:
(3) Something hidden:
(4) Suitability for course:
(5) Interviewer's prognosis:

Chronological Data

PERIOD I   Autumn 1950–Easter 1956

Pre-Selection: Experiments and Testing

1. *Pilot Studies*
   Seminars A to F, October 1950–July 1953
   Balint (with Dicks, Kelnar, Markillie, and Sutherland)

2. *Research* with the 'Old Guard'
   Two parallel seminars, January 1953–April 1955
   Michael and Enid Balint

3. *Testing the Method*
   'Old Guard' combined into one seminar and continued till April 1956
   Seminar G (M. Balint), October 1954–November 1956
   Seminar H (M. Balint), April 1955–August 1957
   Gosling and Turquet join as Associates

PERIOD II April 1956–

Post-Selection: Expansion and Establishment

1. *New Seminars* after introduction of Mutual Selection Interview in April 1956
   Seminar I (M. Balint), April 1956–August 1958

Seminar J (Turquet), October 1956–December 1958
Seminar L (Gosling), May 1957–January 1959
Seminar M (M. Balint), October 1957–November 1961
Seminar N (Turquet), April 1958–July 1960
Seminar O (Gosling), May 1958–July 1959
Seminar P (M. Balint), October 1958–July 1961
Seminar Q (Stauble), October 1958–July 1959
Seminar S (Gosling), October 1959–July 1961
Seminar T (Jacobs), May 1960–July 1962
Seminar U (Turquet), November 1960–July 1963
Seminar V (Goldblatt), October 1961–July 1963
Seminar W (Kelnar), May 1962–July 1964
Seminar X (Gosling), January 1963
Seminar Y (Wilson), November 1963–
Seminar Z (Turquet), November 1964–

2. *Continuation Seminars*

Maintenance Seminar (Kelnar), April 1956–
Reshuffle introduced July 1956
Continuation Seminars taken by all members of staff including Goldblatt from October 1958, Wilson from October 1960, and Bourne from October 1963.

3. *Other Ventures*

Seminar for Hospital Consultants (M. Balint), November 1956–March 1959
Seminar for Registrars (M. Balint), April 1959–July 1960
Research Seminars: Special Problems in General Practice (M. Balint), January 1957–August 1961; (E. Balint), October 1962–
Seminars for Family Planning Association Doctors (M. & E. Balint, Hildebrand, and Friedman), March 1958–July 1963.

κ

4. *The Study of Seminar Technique*
   Associates from other institutions from 1956
   Staff seminars introduced January 1961
   Conferences with Dutch psychiatrists and general
   practitioners, 1959 and 1960
   International Conferences for Seminar Leaders, 1962
   and 1964
   Evaluation of Training Scheme begun August 1961

References

ABRAHAMS, S. I. (1958). 'How to Start and When to Stop'. *J. Coll. Gen. Pract.* **1**, Supp. 2, 25–9.

ABRAHAMS, S. I. (1958). 'Psychological Medicine in General Practice'. *Brit. Med. J.* **2**, 585–90.

BALINT, M. (1954). 'Training General Practitioners in Psychotherapy'. *Brit. Med. J.* **1**, 115–20.

BALINT, M. (1955). 'The Doctor, His Patient and The Illness' (paper). *Lancet*, **1**, 683–8.

BALINT, M. (with ENID BALINT) (1955). 'Dynamics of Training in Groups for Psychotherapy'. *Brit. J. Med. Psych.* **28**, 135–42.

BALINT, M. (1957a). *The Doctor, His Patient and The Illness.* London: Pitman; New York: International Universities Press (2nd edition, enlarged and revised, 1964).

BALINT, M. (1957b). 'Psychotherapy and the General Practitioner'. *Brit. Med. J.* **1**, 156–8.

BALINT, M. (1959). 'Opening Moves in Psychotherapy'. *J. of Hillside Hosp.* **8**, Nos. 1 & 2.

BALINT, M. (1960a). 'The Doctor's Responsibility'. *Med. World*, **92**, 529–35

BALINT, M. (1960b). 'The Marital Problem Clinic – a Problem Child of the F.P.A'. *Family Planning*, **9**, 18–20.

BALINT, M. (1960c). 'Examination by the Patient'. *Excerpta Medica*, International Congress Series, **53**, 9–14.

BION, W. R. (1961). *Experiences in Groups.* London: Tavistock Publications; New York: Basic Books.

135

A Study of Doctors

CLYNE, M. B. (1958). 'The Doctor's Attitude to his Patient'. *Lancet*, 1, 232–6.

CLYNE, M. B. (1960a). 'Läkeren och hands patient' ('The Doctor and his Patient'). *Nytt och Nyttigt* (Sweden), 1, 1.

CLYNE, M. B. (1960b). 'Psychotherapy and the G.P.'. *Med. World* (London), 93, 416–21.

CLYNE, M. B. (1960c). 'Arzt am Schwidewege' ('The Physician at the Crossroads'). *Hessisches Arzteblatt* (Germany), 21, 311.

CLYNE, M. B. (1961). *Night Calls*. London: Tavistock Publications; Philadelphia and Montreal: Lippincott.

CLYNE, M. B. (1964). '30-seconds Psychotherapy'. *Med. World* (London), 100, 9–14.

CLYNE, M. B., HAWES, A. J., LASK, A. & SAVILLE, P. R. (1963). 'The Discontented Patient'. *J. Coll. Gen. Pract.* 6, 87–102.

FAMILY DISCUSSION BUREAU (1955). *Social Casework in Marital Problems. The Development of a Psychodynamic Approach*. London: Tavistock Publications.

FAMILY DISCUSSION BUREAU (1960). *Marriage: Studies in Emotional Conflict and Growth*. London: Methuen.

FAMILY DISCUSSION BUREAU (1962). *The Marital Relationship as a Focus for Casework*. Codicote Press.

HOPKINS, P. (1955). *Modern Trends in Psychosomatic Medicine*. D. O'Neill (Ed.) London: Butterworth.

HOPKINS, P. (1956a). 'Psychotherapy in General Practice'. *Lancet*, 2, 455–7.

HOPKINS, P. (1956b). 'Referrals in General Practice'. *Brit. Med. J.* 2, 873–7.

HOPKINS, P. (1958a). 'Hypertension in General Practice'. *Practitioner*, 180, 463–72.

HOPKINS, P. (1958b). 'The Use of Psychotherapy in General Practice'. *Brit. J. Clin. Pract.* 12, 525–30.

HOPKINS, P. (1959a). 'Gynaecological Disorders in General Practice'. *J. Coll. Gen. Pract.* **2**, 246–51.

HOPKINS, P. (1959b). 'Health and Happiness and the Family'. *Brit. J. Clin. Pract.* **13**, 311–13.

HOPKINS, P. (1959c). 'Menorrhagia in General Practice'. *Med. World* **90**, 531–3.

HOPKINS, P. (1960). 'Psychiatry in General Practice'. *Postgrad. Med. J.* **36**, 323–30.

HORDER, J. (1959). 'How Important are Psychogenic Symptoms?' *Practitioner* **182**, 96–100.

HORDER, J., FINLAY, B., *et al.* (1956). 'The Management of Stress Disorders in General Practice'. *Practitioner* **177**, 729–43.

LASK, A. (in press). 'People with Asthma'. London: Tavistock Publications.

MALAN, D. H. (1963). *A Study of Brief Psychotherapy.* London: Tavistock Publications; Philadelphia and Montreal: Lippincott.

NEWELL, R. R., CHAMBERLAIN, W. E. & RIGLER, L. (1954). 'Descriptive Classification of Pulmonary Shadows'. *Amer. Rev. Tuber.* **69**, 566–84.

PASMORE, S. (1958). 'Psychiatry in General Practice'. *Lancet* **1**, 524–6.

PASMORE, S. (1959). 'The Stabilizing Role of the General Practitioner'. *Brit. J. Clin. Pract.* **13**, 311–13.

RICE, A. K. (1953). 'An Approach to Problems of Labour Turnover'. *Brit. Management Rev.* **2**, 19–47.

SAVILLE, P. R. (1957). 'Psychotherapy and the General Practitioner'. *Brit. Med. J.* **1**, 158–60.

YERUSHAMY, J. (1953). 'Reliability of Chest Roentgenography'. *Dis. of the Chest* **24**, 133–47.

Additional Reading

BALINT, M. (1957). 'Training Medical Students in Psychotherapy. *Lancet*, **2**, 1015–18.

BALINT, M. (1961). 'The other Part of Medicine'. *Lancet*, **1**, 40–2.

BALINT, M. (1961). 'The Pyramid and the Psychotherapeutic Relationship. *Lancet*, **2**, 1051–4.

BALINT, M. & BALINT, E. (1962). *Psychotherapeutic Techniques in Medicine*. London: Tavistock Publications; Philadelphia and Montreal: Lippincott.

BALINT, M. (1965). 'The Doctor's Therapeutic Function'. *Lancet*, **1**, 1177–80.

Index

Index

140

Printed and bound by CPI Group (UK) Ltd, Croydon, CR0 4YY

01/11/2024

01782632-0014